The Communication Disorders Workbook

Designed to help those studying speech–language pathology, this highly useful workbook is both an introduction to the basic concepts and a teaching tool to develop and test students' knowledge. Frequently encountered communication disorders are included, as are conditions less commonly found in speech–language pathology curricula, but which feature increasingly in clinical caseloads.

Features:

- 330 short-answer questions help students to develop knowledge of the causes and features of communication disorders.
- 60 data analysis exercises give students practice in analysing clinical linguistic data.
- Full answers to the exercises are provided, saving the lecturer time in devising responses; students can use the responses to test their own knowledge and understanding.
- A detailed glossary of terms makes the text self-contained, avoiding the need to consult other sources for explanations.
- Suggestions for further reading are provided for each chapter.

Louise Cummings is Professor of Linguistics at Nottingham Trent University. She is a member of the Royal College of Speech and Language Therapists and is registered with the Health and Care Professions Council in the UK.

The Communication Disorders
Workbook

LOUISE CUMMINGS

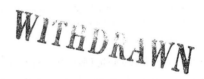
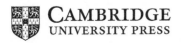
CAMBRIDGE
UNIVERSITY PRESS

CAMBRIDGE
UNIVERSITY PRESS

University Printing House, Cambridge CB2 8BS, United Kingdom

Published in the United States of America by Cambridge University Press, New York

Cambridge University Press is part of the University of Cambridge.

It furthers the University's mission by disseminating knowledge in the pursuit of education, learning and research at the highest international levels of excellence.

www.cambridge.org
Information on this title: www.cambridge.org/9781107633414

© Louise Cummings 2014

First published 2014

Printed in the United Kingdom by Clays, St Ives plc

A catalogue record for this publication is available from the British Library

Library of Congress Cataloguing in Publication data
Cummings, Louise, author.
The communication disorders workbook / Louise Cummings.
   p.   cm.
Includes bibliographical references and index.
ISBN 978-1-107-05498-1 (hardback)
I. Title.
[DNLM: 1. Language Disorders – Case Reports.   2. Language Disorders –
Programmed Instruction.   3. Communication Disorders – Case Reports.
4. Communication Disorders – Programmed Instruction. WL 18.2]
RC428
616.85′506 – dc23   2013037707

ISBN 978-1-107-05498-1 Hardback
ISBN 978-1-107-63341-4 Paperback

Contents

Preface

The clinical education of students in speech and language therapy (SLT) involves a demanding curriculum encompassing knowledge of linguistic and medical disciplines alongside the development of more practically oriented skills. Within this curriculum, there is often little time to develop the analytical skills which SLT students must possess in order to characterize communication disorders. These skills include the ability to characterize the phonetic and phonological processes which underlie disordered speech in cleft palate, the errors in morphosyntax of children with specific language impairment, the impairments in lexical semantics in adults with aphasia, and the pragmatic and discourse anomalies of clients with schizophrenia. The development of these skills is often only possible after many hours of practice in working with actual clinical data. However, the time constraints of most SLT curricula limit the extent to which this level of practical experience can be achieved. It is with a view to resolving this dilemma for clinical educators that this volume has been devised.

This workbook aims to give SLT students extensive practice in identifying and characterizing the full range of communication disorders which are part of the clinical caseload of speech and language therapists. No communication disorder or clinical population is omitted from consideration. Also, impairment or breakdown at each level of linguistic analysis is included, from phonetics, phonology and morphology to syntax, semantics, pragmatics and discourse. Spoken and written language disorders are examined as are aspects of non-verbal communication. Students will learn to characterize expressive and receptive impairments of communication, the clinical features of a range of pathologies with implications for communication and also develop their knowledge of the aetiology of communication disorders. The volume contains 330 short-answer questions and 60 data analysis exercises, each of which poses five questions. So, in total, there are over 600 questions which challenge students on different aspects of communication disorders. All questions are accompanied by answers so that students can check their understanding and monitor their performance. A glossary and suggestions for further reading are additional features of the text which will also facilitate student learning. The glossary is particularly detailed and contains not just communication disorders terminology, but also a range of related clinical terms and expressions.

The titles included in the suggestions for further reading are intended to give the reader a comprehensive background to the various communication disorders which are examined in this workbook. High-level research books and articles have been avoided in preference for material that is suitable for student readers of all stages. Where a specific chapter, section or part is relevant, it is indicated in brackets.

The exercises in this volume have arisen in large part from my teaching of communication disorders and clinical linguistics to university students. In these courses, I have found the short-answer questions to be particularly valuable when used as weekly homework tasks, quizzes in class, and questions for use in examinations. The data analysis exercises are especially effective in small group work in class or in instructor-facilitated classroom discussion. These exercises are also useful when employed as the basis of extended assignments. Students will find the additional practice afforded by these questions and exercises to be excellent preparation for formal assessments. Of course, these uses of the material in this workbook are by no means exhaustive. Instructors and students will no doubt find other ways to use the contents of this volume to good effect in developing knowledge of communication disorders, and the practical skills of linguistic analysis that are needed to characterize those disorders.

Acknowledgements

There are a number of people and organizations whose assistance I wish to acknowledge. I particularly want to thank Dr Andrew Winnard, Commissioning Editor in Language and Linguistics at Cambridge University Press, for responding so positively to the proposal of a workbook in the area of communication disorders. The National Association of Laryngectomy Clubs has once again shown itself to be a strong supporter of any effort which contributes to the clinical education of speech and language therapy students. The association's contribution of the voices of six speakers who have undergone a laryngectomy in Chapter 7 is most gratefully acknowledged. I wish to thank Trevor Pull, Learning Resources Manager at Nottingham Trent University, for his preparation of audio recordings used in Chapter 7. Finally, I have been supported in this endeavour by family members and friends who are too numerous to mention individually. I am grateful to them for their kind words of encouragement during my many months of work on this volume.

Data analysis exercises

Chapter 1

Introduction to communication disorders

Human communication is a complex activity that draws on a diverse set of linguistic, cognitive and motoric skills. These skills are the basis upon which speakers (and writers) generate appropriate communicative intentions, encode and decode linguistic utterances and program and execute the motor movements that are needed to produce those utterances. An understanding of these skills and how they contribute to the formulation and comprehension of linguistic utterances is a prerequisite for the study of communication disorders.

The study of communication disorders also requires an understanding of a number of key clinical distinctions. A communication disorder may have its onset in the developmental period. Alternatively, normally acquired speech and language skills may be disrupted by illnesses and events in late childhood and adulthood. The distinction between a developmental and an acquired communication disorder has implications for all aspects of the management of a communication disorder. Similarly, clinicians recognize a distinction between speech disorders and language disorders and, within language disorders, a distinction between expressive and receptive language impairments. A client may exhibit all of these disorders, or just one.

Clinicians must draw on a range of linguistic and medical disciplines to understand the communication disorders they encounter in clients. Knowledge of phonetics, phonology, morphology, syntax, semantics, pragmatics and discourse is essential for the identification and characterization of all communication disorders (Cummings, 2013a). Similarly, clinicians must have a sound understanding of anatomy, physiology, neurology, psychiatry and ENT medicine (otorhinolaryngology) if they are to understand the medical aetiologies of communication disorders. Aside from linguistic and medical disciplines, clinicians must also be familiar with branches of psychology (e.g. developmental psychology and cognitive psychology) and education in order to assess and treat communication disorders. Each of these disciplines has a part to play in the study of communication disorders and in the clinical management of clients with these disorders.

Section A: Short-answer questions

1.1 Human communication and its disorders

(1) The starting point in the communication of a linguistic message is having a clear communicative _____ that the speaker wants to convey to the hearer.

(2) Which of the following occurs during language encoding?
   (a) Nervous impulses bring about the contraction of muscles that are used in articulation.

(b) The phonological, syntactic and semantic structures that form an utterance are selected.

(c) The auditory centres in the brain recognize nervous impulses as speech sounds.

(d) The speaker forms an idea that he or she wishes to communicate.

(e) A motor plan is constructed.

(3) *True* or *False*: During motor programming, articulators receive nervous impulses instructing them to perform particular movements.

(4) Which of the following occurs during the sensory processing stage of the human communication cycle?

(a) Sound waves are converted by the ear into nervous impulses which are then carried to the auditory centres in the brain.

(b) The brain recognizes certain nervous signals as speech and non-speech sounds.

(c) The articulatory movements that are required to produce an utterance are planned.

(d) A speaker's communicative intention in producing an utterance is established.

(e) The phonological, syntactic and semantic structures that form an utterance are selected.

(5) *True* or *False*: The speech disorders dysarthria and apraxia of speech involve an impairment of motor programming and motor execution, respectively.

(6) In which of the following communication disorders is there a deficit in language decoding?

(a) specific language impairment

(b) developmental verbal dyspraxia

(c) stuttering

(d) acquired dysarthria

(e) selective mutism

(7) In which of the following clinical populations is there difficulty in forming an appropriate communicative intention?

(a) children with cleft lip and palate

(b) adults with Parkinson's disease

(c) adults with schizophrenia

(d) children with developmental stuttering

(e) adults with aphasia

(8) Which of the following clients displays impaired language encoding?

(a) the teacher with vocal nodules

(b) the retired nurse with non-fluent aphasia

(c) the child with developmental verbal dyspraxia

(d) the teenager who stutters

(e) the adult with dysarthria

(9) *True* or *False*: Children and adults with autism spectrum disorders have difficulty in recovering a speaker's communicative intentions.

(10) In which of the following disorders is impaired recognition of spoken words – a condition known as verbal auditory agnosia – to be found?

(a) specific language impairment

(b) developmental phonological disorder

(c) acquired apraxia of speech

    (d) Landau-Kleffner syndrome
    (e) Prader-Willi syndrome

1.2   Significant distinctions in speech-language pathology

(1) Which of the following tasks is assessing a client's receptive syntax?
    (a) A child with Down's syndrome is asked to group pictures into the categories *fruit* and *furniture*.
    (b) An adult with aphasia is asked to name pictures of objects.
    (c) A child with specific language impairment is asked to point to the picture that corresponds to the utterance *The man, who is fat, is climbing the tree.*
    (d) An adult with Williams syndrome is asked to tell a story based on a series of pictures.
    (e) A child with foetal alcohol syndrome is asked to explain the rules of a game to a therapist.

(2) *True* or *False*: The child who says [tat] for *cat* has a problem with expressive phonology.

(3) *True* or *False*: The adult with cerebral palsy who has dysarthria has an acquired communication disorder.

(4) Which of the following clients has a developmental communication disorder?
    (a) an adult with fluent aphasia
    (b) a teenager with persistent stuttering
    (c) an adult with specific language impairment
    (d) a child with foetal alcohol syndrome and language impairment
    (e) an adult with semantic dementia

(5) Which of the following clients has a speech disorder?
    (a) an adult with stroke-induced dysarthria
    (b) a teenager with puberphonia or mutational falsetto
    (c) an adult with auditory agnosia
    (d) a child with developmental verbal dyspraxia
    (e) an adult with anomic aphasia

(6) Fill in the blank spaces in these paragraphs using the words in the box below:
Speech and language therapists who work with clients with communication disorders recognize a number of important clinical distinctions. Depending on when a communication disorder has its onset, it is described as either developmental or _____ in nature. The child who has language impairment in the presence of a genetic syndrome such as _____ X syndrome is described as having a _____ communication disorder. This is because the child's language impairment is related to neurodevelopmental events which have their onset during _____. Alternatively, an adult with previously intact communication skills may sustain a _____ brain injury which results in a speech disorder. The communication impairment in this case is acquired in nature, as the disorder has its onset in _____ when speech skills are fully developed.

    Another significant clinical distinction concerns the difference between a speech disorder and a _____ disorder. Although the lay person is likely to call any communication problem a 'speech disorder', this label is only applied by speech and language therapists to a specific group of communication disorders. Where communication is impaired on account of breakdown in any aspect of the motor planning or _____ of speech, a speech disorder is typically diagnosed. So, the child or adult with hypernasal speech related to _____ incompetence, regardless of the medical aetiology which underlies this incompetence (e.g. cleft _____ or cerebral _____), has a speech disorder. Alternatively, where communication is compromised on account of a failure to manipulate phonological, _____, semantic or pragmatic aspects of language, a language disorder is diagnosed. The child or adult who cannot comprehend sentences which contain a passive _____ construction has a language disorder. This deficit in receptive syntax may arise on account of stroke-induced _____ in the adult or _____ disability in the child with Down's syndrome. This example also demonstrates another important clinical distinction between a receptive and an _____ language disorder. In a _____ language disorder, the comprehension or decoding of an aspect of language is compromised. In an expressive language disorder, the production or _____ of language is impaired. The adult with aphasia who cannot decode a _____ voice construction may also be unable to encode such a construction.

palsy	execution	active	gestation	fragile
velopharyngeal	receptive	decoding	adulthood	
mental	traumatic	lip	voice	language
phonetic	developmental	aphasia	palate	acquired
intellectual	encoding	lexical	hemisphere	
syntactic	expressive	passive	apraxia of speech	

(7) Which of the following clients has an acquired communication disorder?
  (a) the teenager with dysarthria following a road traffic accident
  (b) the adult with frontotemporal dementia and a language impairment
  (c) the child with cleft palate and a phonological disorder
  (d) the teenager with persistent stuttering
  (e) the adult with a brain tumour and apraxia of speech

(8) Which of the following clients has a language disorder?
  (a) an adult with conversion aphonia
  (b) a child with developmental phonological disorder
  (c) a teenager with vocal nodules
  (d) a child with a posterior fossa tumour and word-finding difficulty
  (e) an adult with AIDS dementia complex and pragmatic disorder

(9) *True* or *False*: The adult with Down's syndrome who cannot comprehend sentences which contain relative clauses has an expressive language disorder.

(10) *True* or *False*: The child with paresis of the velum and hypernasality following a traumatic brain injury has a speech disorder.

1.3 Disciplines integral to speech-language pathology

(1) Which of the following medical specialists has primary responsibility for the diagnosis and treatment of vocal fold pathologies?
  (a) neurologist
  (b) otolaryngologist
  (c) psychiatrist
  (d) endocrinologist
  (e) paediatrician

(2) Which of the following linguistic disciplines must the speech and language therapist draw on to characterize problems with inflectional suffixes in children with specific language impairment?
(a) semantics
(b) phonology
(c) morphology
(d) prosody
(e) pragmatics

(3) Which of the following medical disciplines is *not* involved in the management of the child with a cleft lip and palate?
(a) orthodontics
(b) gastroenterology
(c) otolaryngology
(d) neurology
(e) psychiatry

(4) *True or False*: The speech and language therapist must have a sound knowledge of neurology to understand the pathological basis of conditions such as multiple sclerosis and Parkinson's disease.

(5) *True or False*: The speech and language therapist must have a sound knowledge of semantics to understand compensatory articulations in the child with a cleft palate.

(6) Which of the following linguistic disciplines are most important to an understanding of the communication problems of the adult with schizophrenia?
(a) phonetics
(b) discourse
(c) pragmatics
(d) phonology
(e) sociolinguistics

(7) The speech and language therapist may need to seek the professional opinion of an _____ when hormonal factors are believed to play a role in a client's voice disorder.

(8) The speech and language therapist may work alongside a _____ or counsellor in the treatment of clients who stutter.

(9) In the management of the transsexual client, the speech and language therapist is part of a multidisciplinary clinical team which includes social workers and psychologists alongside medical professionals such as _____.

(10) The linguistic discipline which sheds most light on the communication impairments of children with autism spectrum disorders is phonology/syntax/pragmatics (indicate one).

Section B: Clinical scenarios

1.4 Human communication breakdown

The human communication cycle is shown below. It portrays communication as a complex process involving eight stages. Read each of the scenarios presented below. Then decide which of the eight stages in the communication cycle is impaired in the client described. Your answer may include one stage or more than one stage.

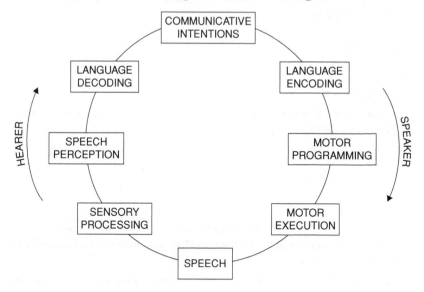

(1) Sally is a sociable 5-year-old who attends primary school. The school's speech and language therapist has assessed Sally's communication skills and has found that her use of phonology is more typical of a 3-year-old child. In all other respects her communication skills are normal.

(2) Bill is 49 years old and has been diagnosed with a brain tumour in his left cerebral hemisphere. Formal assessment of his language skills reveals that his comprehension and production of syntax is disrupted. His speech is also somewhat slurred and mildly unintelligible.

(3) Frank is 65 years old and has been diagnosed with Alzheimer's disease. His participation in conversation has steadily diminished as he has found it increasingly difficult to make relevant contributions to verbal exchanges with others. An assessment of his communication skills reveals relatively intact structural language skills but marked difficulty in generating appropriate messages for communication.

(4) Felicity is 6 years old. She was born with Möbius syndrome which has affected a number of the cranial nerves used in speech production. She is attending regular speech and language therapy where the focus of therapy is on improving the intelligibility of her speech.

(5) Toby is 7 years old and is in recovery following severe bacterial meningitis. The infection has caused bilateral damage to the cochlea in his inner ear. Audiological assessment has revealed significant sensorineural hearing loss. His language skills are age appropriate.

(6) Rose is 50 years old and is two years post-onset a traumatic brain injury that was sustained in a road traffic accident. Her expressive and receptive language skills are relatively intact. However, she has marked difficulty in sequencing the articulatory movements that are needed to produce speech and her vowels are severely distorted. The speech and language therapist diagnoses acquired verbal dyspraxia.

1.5 Clinical distinctions

This exercise is intended to get you thinking about three important distinctions in the study of communication disorders: (1) receptive vs. expressive communication disorders, (2) developmental vs. acquired communication disorders and (3) speech vs. language disorders. Each of the scenarios below examines one of these three distinctions. You need to state which distinction within your answer.

(1) Landau-Kleffner syndrome (LKS) is a rare disorder in children that has a peak incidence between four and seven years of age (Temple, 1997). It leads to sudden or gradual loss of language skills in the presence of a seizure disorder (the children who develop LKS experience seizures as they sleep). Another term for LKS is '*acquired* epileptic aphasia'. Why is the term 'acquired' used of this disorder when it is exclusively children who develop the condition?

(2) Patrick is 59 years old. He is aphasic following a cerebrovascular accident (CVA) some six months earlier. His communication skills have been assessed by a speech and language therapist using the Boston Diagnostic Aphasia Examination (Goodglass et al., 2001), amongst other assessments. This has revealed that Patrick struggles to understand certain syntactic constructions (e.g. relative clauses and passive voice) and that he produces semantic paraphasic errors when asked to name pictures (i.e. his errors are semantically related to the target word, e.g. he says 'eye' for ear). Are Patrick's difficulties with syntax and semantics expressive or receptive in nature?

(3) Penelope is 8 years old and she has a severe communication disorder. Her problems with communication are so severe that she is unable to attend mainstream school and must attend a special school that has a team of speech and language therapists. Penelope's therapist has extensively assessed her communication skills and has noted the following: significant distortion of consonants and vowels, reports of unintelligibility from caregivers and teachers, age-appropriate performance on the Clinical Evaluation of Language Fundamentals (Semel et al., 2003). Does Penelope have a speech disorder, a language disorder or both?

(4) John is 27 years old and has schizophrenia. His communication skills are bizarre which has led to withdrawal and social isolation from everyone other than close family members. Informal observation by a speech and language therapist reveals marked impairment in the pragmatics of language. Specifically, John fails to understand humour and irony used by others and he interprets many utterances literally (e.g. he responds 'yes' to indirect speech acts such as 'Can you tell me the time?'). Also, he contributes many irrelevant utterances in conversation and produces utterances that are poorly related to each other. Are John's problems with pragmatics receptive or expressive in nature?

(5) Frank is 45 years old. He is currently under the supervision of a speech and language therapist who is treating him for a speech disorder (dysarthria) that he developed as a result of a head injury sustained in a motorbike accident. This is not Frank's first contact with speech and language therapy. When he was 5 years old he was diagnosed with grammatical delay by a therapist at the primary school he attended. Frank has experienced two communication disorders to date. Are these disorders developmental or acquired in nature?

(6) Paul is a lively 6-year-old who has a number of cognitive and communication problems caused by his mother's excessive consumption of alcohol during pregnancy (he has been diagnosed as having foetal alcohol syndrome by a paediatrician). His expressive syntax is severely delayed – he is still only at the two-word stage of language production. An analysis of his expressive phonology reveals a number of immature phonological processes. However, his articulation skills are intact. Does Paul have a speech disorder, a language disorder or both?

1.6 Foundational disciplines

The study of communication disorders draws on a diverse knowledge base. Clinicians and researchers must have a sound understanding of a number of linguistic disciplines. However, they must also understand how a range of medical disciplines impact upon this field of work. The statements in (A) below describe linguistic features and errors in a range of child and adult clients. For each statement, name the branch of linguistics (e.g. phonology, syntax) that is used to characterize the feature in question. The statements in (B) below describe different aspects of the medical knowledge that clinicians and researchers draw upon in their work on communication disorders. Name the branch of medicine (e.g. neurology, psychiatry) to which each of these statements relates.

Part A: Linguistics

(1) An aphasic adult is asked by a therapist to describe a picture in which an elderly man is walking a dog. The patient struggles to say 'Man . . . walk . . . dog'.

(2) A 5-year-old child says to his mother 'Can we go in the [tar]?' when he wants to be taken for a drive in the car.

(3) A child with an autism spectrum disorder starts to talk about his friends when he is asked what school he attends.

(4) An adult with Down's syndrome cannot categorize pictures of objects according to the fields *fruit*, *clothing* and *furniture*.

(5) A child with specific language impairment (SLI) says to his teacher 'Bobby make a mess'.

(6) During an articulation test, a child with a cleft palate says [ʔa] for 'cat'.

(7) An analysis of the verbal output of a patient with traumatic brain injury (TBI) reveals a lack of cohesion and extensive repetitiveness.

(8) An adult with aphasia is describing a picture in which a young girl is building a snowman. He says 'She builds a stowcan'.

(9) An adult with autism is asked by a social worker 'Can you close the door?' He responds 'Yes' but does not get up to close the door.

(10) A child with language delay is asked by a therapist to point to a picture in which a girl is being hit by a boy. The child points to a picture showing a girl hitting a boy.

Part B: Medicine

(1) An undersized mandible (micrognathia) is a feature of both Treacher Collins syndrome and Pierre Robin syndrome.

(2) A vocal polyp is detected on the left vocal fold during laryngoscopy.

(3) Following surgical repair of a cleft in the palate, the velum may be insufficiently mobile to achieve the elevation that is needed to make contact with the posterior pharyngeal wall.

(4) If fusion of the maxillary processes does not occur, a child will be born with a cleft in the upper lip.

(5) Aphasia is associated with a lesion in the inferior frontal gyrus (Broca's area) of the left cerebral hemisphere.

(6) Oro-nasal fistulae can appear in the palate after surgical repair of a cleft. Some fistulae can compromise speech production.

(7) A diagnosis of schizophrenia is based on the identification of positive symptoms (e.g. thought disorder) and negative symptoms (e.g. social withdrawal).

(8) In families who have children with SLI, two regions on chromosomes 16 and 19 have been linked to language-related measures.

(9) The facial nerve (cranial nerve VII) innervates the orbicularis oris, the sphincter muscle that encircles the lips.

(10) A patient with hyponasal speech is referred by his general practitioner to the regional hospital for further investigation. Examination of his nasal cavities reveals a well-developed nasal polyp.

SUGGESTIONS FOR FURTHER READING

Atkinson, M. and McHanwell, S. 2002. *Basic medical science for speech and language therapy students*, London and Philadelphia: Whurr.

Black, M. and Chiat, S. 2003. *Linguistics for clinicians: a practical introduction*, London: Arnold.

Cummings, L. 2008. *Clinical linguistics*, Edinburgh: Edinburgh University Press (chapter 1).

    2013a. 'Clinical linguistics: a primer', *International Journal of Language Studies* **7**:2, 1–30.

    2014a. *Communication disorders*, Houndmills: Palgrave Macmillan (chapter 1).

Fogle, P. T. 2013. *Essentials of communication sciences and disorders*, Clifton Park, NY: Delmar (chapter 1).

Justice, L. M. 2010. *Communication sciences and disorders: a contemporary perspective*, second edition, Upper Saddle River, NJ: Pearson (chapter 1).

Morris, D. 2005. *Dictionary of communication disorders*, London: Whurr.

Nicolosi, L., Harryman, E. and Kresheck, J. 2004. *Terminology of communication disorders: speech-language-hearing*, fifth edition, Baltimore and Philadelphia: Lippincott Williams & Wilkins.

Owens Jr, R. E., Metz, D. E. and Farinella, K. A. 2011. *Introduction to communication disorders: a lifespan evidence-based perspective*, fourth edition, Upper Saddle River, NJ: Pearson (chapter 2).

Chapter 2

Developmental speech disorders

For a significant number of children, the acquisition of speech in the developmental period does not occur along normal lines. During embryonic development, a range of craniofacial malformations may occur, leading to structural defects of the anatomical structures which are necessary for speech production. For example, the tissues of the palate and upper lip may fail to fuse during the first trimester of pregnancy, resulting in a cleft of the lip and hard and soft palates. This craniofacial anomaly may occur in isolation or alongside a number of other defects as part of a syndrome (e.g. Pierre Robin syndrome). Other syndromes in which there is abnormal development of the organs of articulation include a small mandible (micrognathia) in Treacher Collins syndrome and abnormal palatal morphology in Down's syndrome. In all these cases, speech acquisition is likely to be compromised to a greater or lesser degree.

Aside from structural defects, the development of speech can also be compromised on account of a neurological impairment. A speech disorder known as dysarthria results when there is damage of the motor centres in the brain and/or any of the pathways which transmit nervous impulses to the muscles of the articulators. The most common cause of developmental dysarthria is cerebral palsy. The child with congenital cerebral palsy has brain damage, often of unknown origin. In cases where the cause of this damage is known, aetiologies can include infections (e.g. maternal rubella), birth anoxia, prenatal exposure to alcohol and cocaine, and traumatic brain injury. Other, less common causes of developmental dysarthria include Duchenne's muscular dystrophy and genetic syndromes (e.g. Down's syndrome). The severity of the speech disorder in dysarthria can range from mild to severe. In the former case, there may be a negligible impact on the intelligibility of speech. In the latter case, speech may be so unintelligible that an alternative means of communication must be found for the client. The child with developmental dysarthria may also have swallowing problems (dysphagia). These problems are also assessed and treated by speech and language therapists.

Another speech disorder which has its onset in the developmental period is developmental verbal dyspraxia (DVD). There is a presumed neurological aetiology of DVD, although a specific brain lesion is rarely identifiable. DVD can be distinguished from developmental dysarthria in a number of ways. In developmental dysarthria, there is neuromuscular weakness which is not present in DVD. Speech errors are also consistent in developmental dysarthria, whereas this is not the case in DVD. The speaker with DVD finds automatic speech production easier than volitional speech production. No such automatic–volitional distinction is evident in the speaker with developmental dysarthria. However, like developmental dysarthria, the speaker with DVD can be highly unintelligible to all but the most familiar hearers.

Section A: Short-answer questions

2.1 Cleft lip and palate

(1) Fill in the blank spaces in these paragraphs using the words in the box below:

A child with a cleft of the palate must overcome a number of structural challenges in his or her production of speech. Even when surgical repair of the cleft has taken place, the _____ may be short and immobile and unable to make contact with the pharyngeal wall. Pulmonary air that is needed for the articulation of oral _____ and fricatives may escape into the _____ cavities. The child may respond to this nasal air escape by engaging in nasal _____ and by shifting the place of articulation of oral sounds. In this way, oral plosives and fricatives may come to be articulated in the _____, where the cleft child is able to establish a build-up of air pressure. The _____ stop [ʔ] may be a common realization of many plosive and fricative sounds. _____ anomalies, including missing teeth and the eruption of teeth in abnormal positions, are common in cleft children and are a further obstacle to speech production. A surgically repaired cleft palate may break down leading to the formation of _____. Some smaller fistulae are asymptomatic, that is, they have no impact on _____ production. The child may attempt to compensate for larger fistulae by shifting the place of articulation back in the _____ tract and by engaging in maladaptive tongue function.

The cleft child's speech production problems are compounded by difficulties with _____. The hearing loss in cleft children is mostly _____ in nature. The function of the _____ tube is to ventilate the middle ear. In the normal ear, this is achieved through the opening of the tube during the contraction of the tensor _____ palatini muscles. These palatal muscles are often abnormal in the cleft child with the result that air fails to enter the _____ ear. In its absence, a condition known as _____ (commonly known as 'glue ear') can develop. The cleft child who is exposed to repeated episodes of otitis media may be deprived of vital speech sound stimulation during critical periods in his or her speech development. To avoid these adverse consequences of otitis media, the cleft child may require the insertion of pressure _____ tubes or 'grommets' in his _____ membrane during a surgical procedure called a _____. It is not unusual for cleft children to require several repetitions of this procedure. As well as surgical intervention, the cleft child will require ongoing audiological assessment to establish hearing levels. Where hearing levels are judged to be inadequate, shorter or longer periods of _____ may be required.

inner	speech	nasal	regurgitation	velum
Reissner's	hearing	glottal	sensorineural	vocal
grimacing	equalizing	middle	tympanic	pharynx
otitis media	dental	plosives	tympanometry	veli
glottis	amplification	otosclerosis	fistulae	audiometry
conductive	Eustachian	palate	myringotomy	turbulence

(2) Which of the following features is associated with cleft lip and palate?
    (a) velopharyngeal incompetence
    (b) micrognathia

     (c) feeding problems

     (d) otitis media

     (e) cholesteatoma

(3) Which of the following is *not* a speech feature of children with cleft palate?

     (a) substitution of oral plosives with glottal stops

     (b) substitution of palato-alveolar fricatives with palatal, velar or pharyngeal fricatives

     (c) a general forward shift in the place of articulation

     (d) the presence of secondary articulations such as nasalization

     (e) hypernasal speech related to velopharyngeal incompetence

(4) *True* or *False*: The embryological malformations that cause cleft lip and palate occur in the second trimester of pregnancy.

(5) *True* or *False*: Audible nasal emissions in children with a cleft palate can mask oral articulations.

(6) Cleft palate is commonly found in infants with Pierre Robin syndrome. Which of the following is *not* associated with this syndrome?

     (a) nasal septum deviation

     (b) micrognathia

     (c) glossoptosis

     (d) microtia

     (e) macroglossia

(7) Which of the following syndromes is associated with cleft lip and palate?

     (a) Möbius syndrome

     (b) Prader-Willi syndrome

     (c) velocardiofacial syndrome

     (d) Down's syndrome

     (e) Asperger's syndrome

(8) In children with a cleft palate, the cleft is surgically repaired in a procedure known as a _____ .

(9) Phonetic defects in the speech of children with a cleft palate can have an adverse effect upon the development of language, and particularly _____ .

(10) *True* or *False*: Electropalatography can be used during therapy with children who have a cleft palate to correct aberrant lingual articulations.

2.2   Developmental dysarthria

(1) Fill in the blank spaces in these paragraphs using the words in the box below:

Children can develop dysarthria in response to a range of cerebral traumas and illnesses. A child may sustain a _____ through a road traffic accident, fall or through physical abuse. An early acquired infection of the central nervous system such as _____ can damage the motor cortices of the brain. A range of prenatal, perinatal and _____ events, a number of which are still poorly understood, can damage the brain's motor centres and result in cerebral _____ . Babies and children can also sustain _____ or strokes, with the resulting cerebral damage giving rise to dysarthria. A degenerative disease such as muscular _____ can cause the muscles of speech production to waste. Children may also develop brain tumours such as posterior _____ tumours. These tumours, as well as the surgery and cranial irradiation that are used to treat them, can damage the cerebral areas that control muscles necessary for speech production. Dysarthria may also be caused by damage to specific _____ nerves. For example, in Möbius syndrome a flaccid dysarthria is caused by bilateral _____ paralysis and VI palsy.

In all these cases, the neural and muscular mechanisms that are necessary for speech production are compromised. The specific effects on speech production of these different events and illnesses can be highly variable and depend to a large extent on the site of _____. For example, if _____ motor neurones are damaged, a spastic dysarthria will result. The child with cerebral palsy frequently exhibits _____ dysarthria, the perceptual features of which are prosodic excess, prosodic insufficiency and articulatory-resonatory incompetence. Spina bifida with hydrocephalus is a neurodevelopmental disorder that involves significant dysmorphology of the cerebellum. Children with this disorder exhibit a number of speech features typical of _____ dysarthria (e.g. articulatory inaccuracy, prosodic excess and phonatory-prosodic insufficiency).

It is important to be aware that a perceived speech feature may be the result of several defective speech production subsystems. For example, words spoken by the dysarthric child may be inappropriately stressed due to poor control of respiration for speech but also due to inefficient valving of the pulmonary airstream during _____. Similarly, the perception that oral consonants are weak may be caused by poor breath control for speech but also by mistiming of the closing of the _____ port (air needed for the production of these consonants may escape through the _____ cavities). To establish which speech production subsystem is primarily responsible for a perceived speech feature, assessment must go beyond perceptual techniques to include _____ and physiological methods as well.

phonation	meningitis	resonation	velopharyngeal	spastic
instrumental	spinal	cerebrovascular accidents		ataxic
traumatic brain injury		hyperkinetic	palsy	cranial
dystrophy	fossa	flaccid	postnatal	lesion
lower	hypokinetic	nasal	upper	facial

(2) Developmental dysarthria can be caused by a range of conditions. Which of the following conditions is associated with this speech disorder?
   (a) Williams syndrome
   (b) Down's syndrome
   (c) Tourette's syndrome
   (d) Worster-Drought syndrome
   (e) Landau-Kleffner syndrome

(3) Which of the following are *true* statements about developmental dysarthria?
   (a) Cerebral palsy is the most common cause of developmental dysarthria.
   (b) Developmental dysarthria only arises from damage to the central nervous system.
   (c) The child with developmental dysarthria also frequently experiences swallowing problems.
   (d) Some forms of developmental dysarthria increase in severity over time.

(e) Oral reflexes, which are suppressed in normally developing children, can persist in children with developmental dysarthria.

(4) A child who has congenital rubella syndrome can present with a mild to moderate dysarthria. The child's speech disorder has been caused by events in the _____ period.

(5) In developmental dysarthria, articulation, _____, resonation, respiration and phonation may all be compromised to varying degrees.

(6) Which of the following statements does *not* describe an aspect of speech production in developmental dysarthria?
(a) Tongue elevation is limited but still adequate for articulatory purposes.
(b) Hypernasal speech is related to velopharyngeal incompetence.
(c) Lip closure for bilabial sounds is impaired.
(d) Jaw movements are aberrant.
(e) Vowels and consonants are distorted.

(7) Which of the following areas are priorities for speech assessment in the child with developmental dysarthria?
(a) the production of non-speech movements of the lips, tongue and velum
(b) the use of respiratory support for speech
(c) the safety of oral feeding
(d) the intelligibility of the child to an unfamiliar listener
(e) the efficiency of velopharyngeal valving of the pulmonary airstream

(8) Which of the following statements are suitable aims of a speech intervention for developmental dysarthria?
(a) the restoration of normal, fully intelligible speech
(b) an improvement in the range and accuracy of tongue movements for speech
(c) the intelligible production of word-initial plosive and fricative consonants
(d) the proficient use of an alternative communication system
(e) the development of strategies to manage drooling, particularly between meals

(9) *True* or *False*: Children with progressive developmental dysarthria can become effective oral communicators.

(10) *True* or *False*: Children with developmental dysarthria display the same inconsistency of speech errors as children with developmental verbal dyspraxia.

2.3 Developmental verbal dyspraxia

(1) Which of the following statements describe features of developmental verbal dyspraxia?
(a) Automatic speech is more adversely affected than volitional speech.
(b) Speech errors are consistent across productions.
(c) Articulation problems are caused by weakness and paralysis of the speech musculature.
(d) Speech errors affect consonants and vowels.
(e) Diadochokinetic rates are within the normal range.

(2) *True* or *False*: Developmental verbal dyspraxia is a motor speech disorder which is more commonly found in girls.

(3) *True* or *False*: The child with developmental verbal dyspraxia displays increasing speech errors with increasing length of words and phrases.

(4) *True* or *False*: The child with developmental verbal dyspraxia often exhibits problems with gross and fine motor skills and has a history of feeding difficulties.

(5) *True* or *False*: The child with developmental verbal dyspraxia exhibits articulatory groping behaviour.

(6) Successful treatment of developmental verbal dyspraxia in children requires an accurate differential diagnosis of the disorder. In diagnosing this disorder, speech and language therapists must attend to:
(a) the presence of a neurological impairment
(b) the types of speech errors that are produced, e.g. substitutions and distortions
(c) the presence of impaired social communication skills
(d) the consistency of speech error production
(e) the child's attentional state and level of cooperation during assessment tasks

(7) Treatment of developmental verbal dyspraxia in children is the subject of much discussion by clinicians. There is general agreement that treatment is most successful when therapy occurs:
(a) on a one-to-one basis with the therapist rather than in a group setting
(b) in longer, less frequent sessions rather than in shorter, more frequent sessions
(c) in an intervention that emphasizes repetitive production and intensive systematic drill
(d) at the same intensity as is recommended for children with a phonological disorder
(e) in shorter, more frequent sessions rather than in longer, less frequent sessions

(8) Children with developmental verbal dyspraxia may _____ their speaking rate as a means of increasing intelligibility.

(9) Select one of the following responses to complete the blank space in the statement: Children with developmental verbal dyspraxia display _____ diadochokinetic rates.
(a) normal
(b) decreased
(c) increased
(d) reduced
(e) inconsistent

(10) Which of the following statements best describes the aetiology of the speech disorder developmental verbal dyspraxia?
(a) The speech disorder has a structural aetiology.
(b) The speech disorder has a neurological aetiology.
(c) The speech disorder has a largely uncertain aetiology although a neurological origin is suspected.
(d) The speech disorder has a mixed structural and neurological aetiology.
(e) The speech disorder has a psychological aetiology.

Section B: Data analysis exercises

2.4   Cleft lip and palate 1

Background

Louise is a young Dutch girl aged 3 years 8 months who was studied by Van Lierde et al. (2000). She has Kabuki make-up syndrome. Her cognitive functioning is normal. She has a submucous cleft palate, a history of otitis media and some hypotonia.

Speech production

Phonetic inventory: Louise could correctly produce all Dutch vowels and 68% of Dutch consonants. She could not produce correctly the nasal [ɲ] and the fricatives [f], [v], [ʃ], [ʒ] and [h].

   Phonotactic analysis: Target syllables were usually retained. A change in syllable structure occurred in only 10% of words.

   Phonetic analysis: Compared to target productions at the segmental level, 55% of Louise's consonants were in error and 21% of her vowels. Consonant errors included omissions, substitutions, distortions and additions. Substitutions were the most common error type. The most common types of distortion errors were dentalization, labiodentalization, devoicing, weak articulation, mild to moderate hypernasality and moderate nasal emission. Vowel errors included lowering, backing, neutralization (replacement by a schwa) and unrounding of a target rounded vowel.

   Phonological process analysis: Syllable structure processes are present including cluster reduction (affecting /s/-, /t/- and /R/-blends), final and initial consonant deletion (the former chiefly affecting final /k/) and deletion of unstressed syllables. The following substitutions were in evidence, some of which are shown in the table below:

(a) /p/ → /f/; /b/ → /v/; /k/ → /X/; /k/ → /s/; /t/ → /f/
(b) /s/ → /t/; /z/ → /b/
(c) /k/ → /t/; /ɣ/ → /p/
(d) /f/ → /j/

Dutch word	English word	Phonemic norm	Client production
sigaret	cigarette	/siˠaRɛt/	[sizaRɛt]
boekentas	satchel	/bukəntas/	[pupətas]
fiets	bicycle	/fits/	[sis]
kapstok	clothes hanger	/kapstɔk/	[tatɔk]
zwart	black	/zwart/	[vat]
gieter	watering-pot	/ˠitər/	[Ritə]
kraan	tap	/kra:n/	[ka:n]
kruis	cross	/krœYs/	[Xœys]
worsten	sausages	/wɔrstən/	[wəs]
borstal	brush	/bɔrstəl/	[bɔtəl]
wolken	clouds	/wɔlkən/	[wɔk]
jongen	boy	/jɔŋən/	[ɔŋə]
kop	head	/kɔp/	[tap]
klok	clock	/klɔk/	[slɔk]

Exercise 1 Louise's speech production displays mild to moderate hypernasality and moderate nasal emission. Which feature(s) of her clinical presentation might explain this articulatory deviance?

Exercise 2 Which phonological processes are exemplified by the substitutions in (a) to (d) above? Which of these processes occur in 'kruis' and 'kop' in the table?

Exercise 3 Give <u>one</u> example of each of the following phonological processes in the above data:

(a) progressive assimilation
(b) regressive assimilation
(c) metathesis
(d) syllable deletion
(e) final consonant deletion.

Exercise 4 What feature do the following productions have in common?

(a) word-initial /kr/ in 'tap' and 'cross'
(b) word-medial /rst/ in 'sausages' and 'brush'
(c) final syllable /ən/ in 'clouds' and 'boy'
(d) word-initial /k/ in 'head' and 'clock'

Exercise 5 Two phonological processes are evident in each of the following productions. State what these processes are in each case.

(a) 'worsten' /wəs/
(b) 'wolken' /wɔk/
(c) 'jongen' /ɔŋə/

2.4 Cleft lip and palate 2

Background

Rachel is a 6-year-old girl who was studied by Howard (1993). She was born 11 weeks prematurely with a central cleft of the hard and soft palates. She underwent cleft repair at 2;2 years. Rachel has a severe speech disorder, but her receptive and expressive language appears to have developed normally. Rachel has a history of fluctuating mild to moderate conductive hearing loss. Grommets were first inserted at 3;0 years and again at 4;0 years. At 5;11 years, T-tubes were inserted. At the time of this study, Rachel had received three years of speech therapy during which time little progress had been made.

Phonotactic structure: glasses [ˈɴwæç̬ɔ̬ç̬] string [ˈfŋʔwɪɴ] matches [ˈmaʔjə̬h̬]

Oral–nasal contrast

letter	[ˈɰeʔə]	nose	[ɴəʊç̬]
ladder	[ˈɰæʔə]	ring	[ʊɪɴ]
sugar	[ˈç̬ʊʔə]	fine	[f̩:aɪɴ]
down	[ʔaʊɴ]	penny	[ˈp͡ʔeɴɪ]
dog	[ʔɒʔʰ]	singing	[ˈç̬ɪɴɪɴ]
cat	[ʔæʔʰ]	teaspoon	[ˈʔiç̬bʊɴ]

Bilabials

pig	[ʘɪʔʰ]	mud	[məʔʰ]
pen	[ʔeɴ]	mum	[məm]
tap	[ʔæʔⵔ]	mouth	[mauʋ]
paper	['p͡ʔeɪp͡ʔə]	thumb	[ʋʋm]
big	[mɪʔʰ]	jam	[ʔjæm]
baby	['ɓeɪbɪ]	hammer	['ħæmə]
bike	[maɪʔʰ]/[ɓaɪʔʰ]		

Stop-fricative-approximant continuum and stop-affricate continuum

tap	[ʔæʔʰ]	zip	[ʑɪʔⵔ]
down	[ʔauɴ]	cup	[ʔʊʔʰ]
chair	[ʔjɛə]	go	[ʔəʊ]
jam	[ʔjæm]	yes	[jɛʔ]
sock	[ʑɒʔʰ]	why	[waɪ]
shop	[ʑjɒp͡ʰ]		

Place of articulation

baby	[ɓeɪbɪ]	bucket	['ɓʊʔɪʔʰ]
toy	[ʔɔɪ]	Sue	[ʑu]
cat	[ʔæʔʰ]	daddy	['ʔæʔɪ]
tap	[ʔæʔⵔ]	dog	[ʔɒʔʰ]
paper	[p͡ʔeɪp͡ʔə]	sugar	['ʑʊʔə]
kick	[ʔɪʔʰ]	shoe	[ʑu]

Voicing

pig	[ʘɪʔʰ]	bib	[ɓɪɓʰ]
baby	['ɓeɪbɪ]	tea	[ʔi]
letter	['ɰeʔə]	ladder	['ɰæʔə]
Sue	[ʑu]	zoo	[ʑu]
watch	[wɒʔʑ]	jam	[ʔjæm]
four	[fɔ]	a van	[ə 'fæɴ]
feather	['feʋə]	laughing	['æfɪɴ]
dig	[ʔɪʔʰ]	chair	[ʔjɛə]
key	[ʔi]	fridge	[fʊɪʔħ]
go	[ʔəʊ]	cover	['ʔʊʋə]

Exercise 1 Is Rachel able to observe the phonotactic structure of targets in her spoken productions? Rachel is able to maintain a broad oral–nasal contrast in her spoken productions. How does she achieve this in the case of alveolar and velar segments?

Exercise 2 How does Rachel achieve an oral–nasal contrast in the case of bilabial segments?

Exercise 3 Does Rachel successfully signal a contrast between stop, fricative and approximant sounds? How does she achieve this contrast? How does she signal a contrast between stops and affricates?

Exercise 4 Prior to therapy, alveolar and postalveolar fricatives had pharyngeal realizations in Rachel's spoken output. Is Rachel now able to signal an alveolar–postalveolar contrast? How does Rachel signal a contrast between bilabial and other plosives?

Exercise 5 Does Rachel observe a voicing contrast for bilabial, alveolar and velar plosives? How does she signal a phonological contrast between /f/ and /v/?

2.5 Developmental dysarthria

Background

The following data are from a child called Mike who was studied by Harris and Cottam (1985). Mike was 4;11 years of age at the time of data collection. He was born one month prematurely and has a congenital heart lesion which has necessitated long periods of hospitalization. Mike has no structural abnormalities of the lips and tongue. However, at rest both structures appear lax: the lips are parted and the tongue tip protrudes slightly. The same general laxness is evident when Mike performs movements during non-verbal tasks. On the basis of these findings, it was concluded that developmental dysarthria is a major contributory factor in Mike's speech unintelligibility.

An articulation test was performed and yielded the following data for analysis. Three features of the south Yorkshire urban vernacular to which Mike is exposed should not be attributed significance within the analysis: (1) the presence of 'h-dropping' (the absence of historical /h/ in words such as 'house'); (2) monophthongal realizations of the nuclei in words such as 'nice' (/aɪ/→ [æ]); and (3) the loss of historical /r/ in preconsonantal and prepausal position (south Yorkshire vernacular is non-rhotic), e.g. 'horsie', 'chair'.

Target	Client production	Target	Client production
boat	[boː?s̪]	paper	[pʰeːɸə]
bottle	[bɒs̪ʊ]	penny	[ɸɛli]
brush	[bəs̪]	pin	[pɸɪn]
cake	[kʰeː?s̪]	pool	[pɸuː]
car	[kʰɑː] ~ [xɑː]	sail	[s̪eːʊ]
cat	[kʰaʔs̪]	sew	[s̪oː]
chair	[ts̪ɛː]	smoke	[moː?s̪]
chimney	[s̪ɪns̪ɪ]	sock	[s̪ɒʔs̪]
cotton	[kxɒs̪ən]	sugar	[s̪əs̪ə]
cuff	[xəf] ~ [kxəf]	tail	[s̪eːʊ]
fin	[fɪn]	tea	[ts̪iː]
hiss	[ɪs̪]	teeth	[tʰiːs̪]
hit	[ɪʔs̪]	three	[fʊiː]
house	[aʊs̪]	toe	[s̪oː]
marching	[mɑːs̪ɪn]	watch	[wɒʔs̪]

(cont.)

Target	Client production	Target	Client production
matches	[maʂə]	water	[wɔːʂə]
milk	[mɪʊx]	night	[næːʔʂ]
nice	[næːʂ]	nothing	[nəʂɪn]
hoof	[uːf]	hoop	[uːpʰ] ~ [uːpɸ]
horsie	[ɔːʂɪ]		

Exercise 1 Mike's speech displays considerable cluster reduction and fronting, the latter of palatoalveolar and velar sounds. Give two examples of cluster reduction, palato-alveolar fronting and velar fronting in the data. Does palatoalveolar and velar fronting occur in all word positions?

Exercise 2 Mike has difficulty producing alveolar and dental fricatives. How are these sounds realized in Mike's speech?

Exercise 3 Mike's speech contains a number of deviant articulatory features which are not seen in either adult speech or as part of normal development. Two of these features are shown below. Give three examples of each of these realizations. Your examples should include realizations in word-initial, word-medial and word-final position. The use of affricates or fricatives for voiceless plosives is the reverse of a pattern seen in normal development. What is that pattern?

(a) voiceless plosives → affricates or fricatives
(b) affricates → fricatives

Exercise 4 In some of Mike's single-word productions, a developmentally normal feature combines with a deviant articulatory feature. This is evident in Mike's production of 'smoke' as [moːʔʂ]. What two articulatory features (one normal, the other deviant) characterize the production of word-final /k/ in 'smoke'?

Exercise 5 Mike also makes use of heavily aspirated plosives in word-initial position. The tendency in Mike's local northern English vernacular is for voiceless plosives to be unaspirated. Give three examples of this feature in the data. Then summarize the three ways in which voiceless plosives and affricates are realized in Mike's speech.

2.6 Developmental verbal dyspraxia

Background

Developmental verbal dyspraxia is a controversial disorder which is found in children. The disorder is also known by the terms 'developmental apraxia of speech (DAS)' and 'childhood apraxia of speech'. In all cases, there is substantial impairment in the production of speech sounds in the absence of evident neurological impairment.

Data 1

The following productions are a sample of the repeated token data collected from three English-speaking male children with developmental apraxia of speech (Marquardt et al., 2004). These children were assessed using articulation testing and spontaneous speech sampling at one-year intervals between the ages of 4;6 and 7;7 years.

Gloss	Target	Token 1	Token 2	Token 3	Token 4
cat	/kæt/	/kæt/	/kɛt/	/kæt/	/kit/
plate	/pleɪt/	/peɪt/	/pɛt/	/pleɪ/	
dog	/dag/	/dag/	/dag/	/dag/	/dag/
chair	/ʧeɪr/	/teɪr/	/teɪr/	/teɪr/	

Data 2

The following table contains the spoken productions of a boy called Ryan with developmental verbal dyspraxia. Ryan is 8 years 8 months old and was studied by McNeill and Gillon (2011).

Target	Client production	Target	Client production
rain	/weɪn/	kangaroo	/dæŋəru/
girl	/dal/	shark	/zak/
teeth	/tif/	fish	/fɪʃ/
chips	/zɪps/	dinosaur	/daɪndɔ/
bridge	/weʤ/	cake	/deɪk/

Exercise 1 What feature of DAS is exemplified by the repeated tokens of 'cat and 'plate' in Data 1? Characterize the speech errors in both cases.

Exercise 2 Describe how the repeated token data for 'dog' and 'chair' differ from the repeated token data for 'cat' and 'plate'.

Exercise 3 In Data 2, some of Ryan's spoken productions contain developmental errors which would be more typical of a younger child. Give three examples of such errors.

Exercise 4 When Ryan makes sound substitutions, is he consistent or inconsistent in the substitutions he makes? Give examples from Data 2 to support your answer.

Exercise 5 Children with developmental verbal dyspraxia also produce vowel errors. Not infrequently, these errors include the realization of diphthongs as monopthongs. Is this a feature of Ryan's speech? Use data to support your answer.

SUGGESTIONS FOR FURTHER READING

Campbell, T. and Gretz, S. A. 2009. 'Apraxia of speech in childhood', in M. R. McNeil (ed.), *Clinical management of sensorimotor speech disorders*, second edition, New York: Thieme, 295–7.

Cummings, L. 2008. *Clinical linguistics*, Edinburgh: Edinburgh University Press (sections 2.2, 2.3 and 4.2).

2014a. *Communication disorders*, Houndmills: Palgrave Macmillan (chapter 2).

Gillam, R. B., Marquardt, T. P. and Martin, F. N. 2011. *Communication sciences and disorders: from science to clinical practice*, second edition, Sudbury, MA: Jones and Bartlett Publishers (chapter 8).

Hodge, M. 2014. 'Developmental dysarthria', in L. Cummings (ed.), *Cambridge handbook of communication disorders*, Cambridge: Cambridge University Press, 26–48.

Love, R. J. 2000. *Childhood motor speech disability*, second edition, Boston: Allyn and Bacon (chapters 1, 3, 4 and 5).

McNeill, B. 2014. 'Developmental verbal dyspraxia', in L. Cummings (ed.), *Cambridge handbook of communication disorders*, Cambridge: Cambridge University Press, 49–60.

Peterson-Falzone, S. J., Hardin-Jones, M. A. and Karnell, M. P. 2010. *Cleft palate speech*, St. Louis, MO: Mosby Elsevier (chapter 7).

Riski, J. E. 2014. 'Cleft lip and palate and other craniofacial anomalies', in L. Cummings (ed.), *Cambridge handbook of communication disorders*, Cambridge: Cambridge University Press, 3–25.

Russell, J. 2013. 'Orofacial anomalies', in J. S. Damico, N. Müller and M. J. Ball (eds.), *The handbook of language and speech disorders*, Oxford: Wiley-Blackwell, 474–96.

Chapter 3

Developmental language disorders

For many children, the acquisition of language does not follow a normal developmental course. For the child with developmental phonological disorder (DPD), the simplification processes which are found in immature speech do not resolve spontaneously as they do in typically developing children. As a result, the child with DPD may persist in using forms such as [tat] for 'cat' (fronting), [peɪn] for 'plane' (consonant cluster reduction), and [dɔ] for 'dog' (final consonant deletion) beyond the chronological age at which these phonological processes normally resolve. Often, there is no clear reason why phonological immaturities and deviances persist, and the child displays normal development in other language and non-language areas.

The child with specific language impairment (SLI) may also have phonological problems, but will additionally present with severe deficits in morphosyntax and semantics. These deficits are not related to hearing loss, emotional disturbance, intellectual disability or any of the other factors which are known to predispose a child to language disorder. Moreover, the developmental delay is specific to language, with performance in other areas within the normal range. A subgroup of children with SLI has significant deficits in pragmatics and is labelled as having 'pragmatic language impairment'.

Aside from DPD and SLI, children can have language disorder as a result of intellectual disability. Often, this is in the context of a genetic syndrome such as fragile X syndrome and Williams syndrome. In such cases, not all aspects of language may be impaired to a similar extent. For example, the child with Down's syndrome has marked impairments in expressive syntax while pragmatics is an area of relative strength. The child with autism spectrum disorder can also present with language impairments. In severe cases, language may never emerge. Where language is acquired, marked pragmatic and discourse impairments may occur alone or alongside structural language deficits (see Cummings (2012) for discussion). The child who sustains a traumatic brain injury may struggle to conduct a conversation, narrate a story or explain the rules of a game to a listener. These communication difficulties may be related to cognitive deficits more than to any impairment of structural language, although the latter may also be present. Finally, the child with a seizure disorder (epilepsy) can exhibit language and communication problems which have an insidious or sudden onset. A severe regression in language skills, such as occurs in the rare disorder Landau-Kleffner syndrome, can leave a child in a state of mutism.

Section A: Short-answer questions

3.1 Developmental phonological disorder

(1) Which of the following statements is *true* of developmental phonological disorder in children?

(a) There is a reduced system of sound contrasts in phonologically disordered children.

(b) The child with phonological disorder has weakness of the articulatory muscles.

(c) Hearing loss explains speech errors in phonologically disordered children.

(d) The phonological processes that occur in children with phonological disorder resolve spontaneously.

(e) Children with phonological disorder always devoice word-initial consonants.

(2) A child with developmental phonological disorder says [toʊm] for 'comb', [peɪn] for 'plane' and [paɪ] for 'fly'. Which of the following statements captures this child's speech errors?

(a) The child exhibits a phonological process called consonant cluster reduction.

(b) The child exhibits gliding and final consonant deletion.

(c) The child exhibits a phonological process called stopping.

(d) The child exhibits velar fronting, consonant cluster reduction and stopping.

(e) The child exhibits vowel errors as well as consonant errors.

(3) *True* or *False*: The phonologically disordered child who says [rɪŋ] for 'string' exhibits the phonological process of consonant cluster reduction.

(4) *True* or *False*: The phonologically disordered child who says [bɪn] for 'pin' exhibits the phonological process of prevocalic devoicing.

(5) *True* or *False*: Male children with developmental phonological disorder outnumber female children with the disorder by approximately 3 to 1.

(6) Which of the following statements is *not* true of the speech sound errors made by children with developmental phonological disorder?

(a) Speech sound errors can be analysed in terms of distinctive features and phonological processes.

(b) Some speech sound errors affect syllable structure, e.g. final consonant deletion.

(c) Only children with developmental phonological disorder engage in processes such as fronting and stopping.

(d) The child who says [gɔg] for 'dog' is engaging in velar assimilation.

(e) Speech sound errors are not related to neuromuscular deficits.

(7) In developmental phonological disorder, consonants are often severely disordered in the presence of an intact _____ system.

(8) Many clinicians subscribe to the view that sounds which are not _____ are poor initial targets for phonological therapy.

(9) Which of the following features distinguishes the child with developmental phonological disorder from the child in which sound simplifications are part of a normal maturational process?

(a) persistence of normal processes

(b) presence of a chronological mismatch in the child's phonological errors

(c) the presence of cluster reduction and final consonant deletion

(d) the presence of unusual, idiosyncratic or atypical processes

(e) the presence of velopharyngeal incompetence

(10) *True* or *False*: Children with a preschool history of developmental phonological disorder have an elevated risk of language and literacy difficulties during the school years.

3.2 Specific language impairment

(1) Which of the following statements characterize specific language impairment (SLI) in children?

 (a) Phonology is uniquely deviant in children with SLI, while morphosyntax is an area of strength.

 (b) Children with SLI exhibit more severe deficits of receptive language than expressive language.

 (c) Cognitive deficits have been linked to language problems in children with SLI.

 (d) Children with SLI can use a 'probable event' strategy to decode reversible passive sentences.

 (e) Children with SLI have poor socialization skills and avoid interaction with others.

(2) Fill in the blank spaces in this paragraph using the words in the box below:
There is a significant group of children in whom language impairment occurs in the absence of a known _____. Specifically, these children lack any neurological basis for their language disorder and have no _____ loss or psychiatric disturbance. Because their impairment is specific to language (i.e. all other areas of development are within the normal range), their disorder is called _____ language impairment. Children with this language disorder usually display marked impairments of _____ and semantics. For example, they may omit _____ morphemes on verbs (e.g. 'He walk very slowly') and nouns (e.g. 'You got two biscuit'). They may fail to invert the subject pronoun and _____ verb in questions (e.g. 'What we can eat?') and may use _____ pronouns instead of subject pronouns (e.g. 'Him drinking juice?'). The comprehension of these different forms may also be impaired. Word learning and lexical _____ abilities are also compromised in children with SLI. While structural language deficits have long been recognized in children with SLI, _____ has traditionally been viewed as an area of relative strength in this clinical population. Alternatively, when pragmatic deficits have occurred, they have been judged to be _____ to problems with language form. However, recent research is revealing that both positions may be mistaken.

derivational	pragmatics	lexical	aetiology
phonology	semantic	hearing	auxiliary
inflectional	object	secondary	discourse
specific	visual	syntax	access and retrieval

(3) *True* or *False*: Children with SLI have less difficulty with the progressive inflection *–ing* than other verb-related morphology.

(4) *True* or *False*: Children with SLI exhibit more severe pragmatic deficits than children with autism spectrum disorders.

(5) The utterance *Her painting* is produced by a child of 3;11 years who has SLI. This child is using the incorrect _____ and has omitted an _____ verb.

(6) Children with SLI display problems with _____ -marking morphemes.

(7) Which of the following conditions precludes a diagnosis of SLI?

(a) the presence of a craniofacial anomaly in a child

(b) the presence of cerebral palsy in a child

(c) the presence of developmental dyslexia in a child's biological relatives

(d) recent episodes of otitis media with effusion in a child

(e) the presence of restricted interests and impaired reciprocal social interaction in a child

(8) Which of the following are *true* statements about the epidemiology of SLI?

(a) SLI is more prevalent in males than in females of all ages.

(b) There is an increased prevalence of SLI in children of lower socioeconomic classes.

(c) The greater prevalence of SLI in males only obtains for children under 5 years of age.

(d) There is an increased prevalence of SLI in children born to mothers with no university education.

(e) The prevalence of SLI in males and females between 5 and 10 years of age is not markedly different.

(9) *True* or *False*: There is an increased prevalence of language impairments in the biological relatives of children with SLI.

(10) In order to receive a diagnosis of SLI, a child must have language test scores _____ standard deviations or more below the mean for their chronological age and a performance IQ of _____ or higher.

3.3 Developmental dyslexia

(1) Which of the following are *true* statements about developmental dyslexia?

(a) Reading difficulties cannot be attributed to a lack of instruction, emotional disorders or sensory disorders.

(b) Developmental dyslexia is of neurobiological origin.

(c) Phonological processing deficits are a common cognitive impairment.

(d) Children with developmental dyslexia seldom exhibit poor spelling.

(e) Children with developmental dyslexia have normal intelligence.

(2) *True* or *False*: The prevalence of developmental dyslexia is higher in girls than in boys in school-referred populations.

(3) Which of the following is *not* an outcome of developmental dyslexia?

(a) increased risk of suicide

(b) increased risk of school drop out

(c) increased risk of psychotic illness

(d) increased risk of incarceration

(e) increased risk of bipolar disorder

(4) Fill in the blank spaces in this paragraph using the words in the box below:

The hallmark phenotype of dyslexia includes problems in phonological and _____ coding, pseudoword reading, _____, inhibition, rapid naming and rapid _____ switching. This phenotype distinguishes children with developmental dyslexia from children with other neurological or _____ disorders which can affect literacy development. For example, difficulties in legible letter _____ , rapid finger tapping tasks and orthographic coding are found in children with _____ only, while problems in oral language and the comprehension of text are found in children with _____ and written language disorders.

oral	dyspraxia	writing	spelling
semantic	orthographic	chromosomal	automatic
developmental	phonics	dysgraphia	cognitive

(5) Which of the following is a purported cause of developmental dyslexia?
    (a) theory of mind deficits
    (b) poor memory
    (c) global problems in automatizing skills
    (d) phonological processing difficulties
    (e) difficulty processing visual information efficiently

(6) *True* or *False*: Phonological processing is not predictive of success in early reading.

(7) *True* or *False*: Deficits in working memory have been identified in children and adults with dyslexia.

(8) Why can researchers not base conclusions about dyslexia in other languages on the example of English?

(9) Which of the following are early risk factors for developmental dyslexia?
    (a) family history of dyslexia
    (b) a sibling with an autism spectrum disorder
    (c) vocabulary deficits
    (d) family history of hearing loss
    (e) letter knowledge deficits

(10) *True* or *False*: Dyslexia in languages with more consistent orthographies than English is characterized by problems in fluency and not in accuracy.

3.4   Intellectual disability

(1) Which of the following conditions is *not* associated with intellectual disability?
    (a) fragile X syndrome
    (b) meningitis
    (c) birth anoxia
    (d) specific language impairment
    (e) phenylketonuria

(2) Which of the following aetiologies of intellectual disability is genetic in nature?
    (a) maternal rubella
    (b) Williams syndrome
    (c) lead exposure
    (d) Prader-Willi syndrome
    (e) cranial irradiation

(3) Which of the following aetiologies of intellectual disability is an infectious disease?
   (a) toxoplasmosis
   (b) Down's syndrome
   (c) encephalitis
   (d) head injury
   (e) cri du chat syndrome

(4) Prenatal alcohol exposure is responsible for language disorder and intellectual disability in children with _____.

(5) *True* or *False*: In children with intellectual disability, the rate of lexical acquisition is markedly delayed.

(6) *True* or *False*: An intelligence quotient (IQ) below 70 is indicative of intellectual disability.

(7) *True* or *False*: In children and adults with genetic syndromes, language skills are always commensurate with mental age.

(8) Which of the following statements capture the language skills of children with Down's syndrome?
   (a) There are significant impairments in expressive syntax.
   (b) Receptive language skills are superior to expressive language skills.
   (c) Pragmatic language skills are superior to structural language skills.
   (d) Phonology is relatively intact in children with Down's syndrome.
   (e) Lexical semantic skills are markedly delayed.

(9) *True* or *False*: Augmentative and alternative communication is not a suitable intervention for children with intellectual disability.

(10) The good visual and motor skills of children with _____ are generally credited with explaining these children's successful use of manual signs such as the Makaton vocabulary.

3.5   Autism spectrum disorder

(1) Fill in the blank spaces in these paragraphs using the words in the box below:
There is a large and growing number of children who have language and communication problems as part of an autism spectrum disorder (ASD). These children are predominantly male. Children with ASD have deficits in more than one area of functioning. To capture this impaired functioning across a number of domains, the diagnostic label _____ developmental disorder is used by clinicians. The language and communication problems of children with ASD are quite unlike those observed in most children that are seen by speech and language therapists. When language does emerge in these children – and in many individuals with autism, particularly those with intellectual disability, it does not – it is markedly deviant in areas that are identified as _____ in nature. These children are less likely than their normally developing peers to initiate _____, respond appropriately to the conversational _____ of others, use gesture and understand the illocutionary _____ of a speaker's utterances. Their spoken output is often echolalic, may display pronoun reversal and is frequently noteworthy on account of its gross _____ disturbances (e.g. inappropriate stress on words and excessive volume).

Children with ASD are particularly poor at understanding the emotional states of others and struggle in particular to use ———— expressions to this end. This failure of social ———— may lead them to misinterpret the remarks of others. For example, it is frequently commented that children with autism respond poorly to the teasing behaviour of other children. One prominent theory of these various deficits in autism locates the central cognitive impairment in a failure to develop a theory of one's own and other minds. These children, it is claimed, are unable to attribute beliefs and other ———— to their own minds and to the minds of others. This theory has considerable plausibility as far as the pragmatic deficits of autism are concerned. The child with autism who is unable to attribute beliefs to a speaker is unable to make predictions about what that speaker intends to communicate by means of producing an utterance. For example, he or she is unable to appreciate that the speaker who utters 'Can you put those toys back in the cupboard?' is not asking a ———— about the child's ability to do something. Rather, the speaker's intention in producing the utterance is to ———— that the child put the toys in the cupboard.

mental states	conversation	request	specific
maxims	pragmatic	pervasive	cognition
prosodic	question	phonetic	turns
speech act	facial	communicative intentions	force

(2) *True* or *False*: The expression 'triad of impairments' refers to deficits in interaction, socialization and imagination in ASD.

(3) *True* or *False*: Approximately 50% of individuals with autistic disorder do not develop functional speech.

(4) *True* or *False*: Pragmatic deficits in ASD are related to theory of mind deficits.

(5) Which of the following are *true* statements about ASD?
  (a) Intelligence quotient (IQ) is always within the normal range.
  (b) Better case ascertainment has led to an increase in the number of diagnosed cases.
  (c) Structural language skills are invariably intact in children and adults with ASD.
  (d) Prosodic deficits can compromise communication in ASD.
  (e) Social functioning is typically in the normal range in ASD.

(6) Which of the following statements characterize the language and communication skills of individuals with ASD?
  (a) Phonology and prosody are both markedly deviant, particularly in children.
  (b) While verbal communication skills are deviant, nonverbal communication skills are age-appropriate.
  (c) Infants with autism display normal prelinguistic communication skills.
  (d) For those children with ASD who become verbal communicators, language skills are most deviant at the level of pragmatics.
  (e) Children with autism can be taught how to use augmentative and alternative communication systems such as the Picture Exchange Communication System.

(7) Which of the following statements does *not* capture a behavioural deficit in autism?

    (a) Children with autism exhibit a cognitive processing style that is characterized by weak central coherence.

    (b) The socialization impairment in autism is manifested in a failure to develop age-appropriate social relationships.

    (c) Children with autism exhibit executive function deficits.

    (d) Children with autism display restricted, repetitive and stereotyped patterns of behaviour, interests and activities.

    (e) Children with autism exhibit deviant verbal and nonverbal communication skills.

(8) *True* or *False*: Communication is the least impaired area of functioning in children and adults with ASD.

(9) Theory of mind (ToM) describes the cognitive ability to attribute mental states to one's own mind and to the minds of others. ToM skills in children with autism are assessed through the use of _____ tests.

(10) *True* or *False*: Children with autism are around 10 years of age before they can pass the same tests of false belief which normally developing children pass at 4 years of age.

3.6 Childhood traumatic brain injury

(1) *True* or *False*: A brain injury in children may be either congenital or acquired.

(2) *True* or *False*: Open head injury represents the largest aetiological category of acquired brain injury in children.

(3) Fill in the blank spaces in these paragraphs using the words in the box below:

A closed head injury (CHI) is a non-penetrating injury to the brain in which the skull and/or dura remain _____. It may result in a number of immediate neuropathological changes. The nerve fibres which make up the _____ matter of the brain are often stretched and rotated by the force of the injury, leading to diffuse _____ damage. Small and large blood vessels may rupture resulting in _____ throughout the brain. Additionally, the brain is not just bruised and lacerated at the point of contact, but also at distant points on account of the brain ricocheting against the _____ protuberances on the inside of the skull. The bony shelves of the anterior and middle fossa place the surfaces of the _____ and temporal lobes at particular risk of this injury. Aside from these immediate effects, there are also secondary effects of CHI. The presence of _____ can cause generalized compression of the brain. A subdural _____ may develop, and intracerebral haemorrhage and localized infarction may occur. Cerebral infections, particularly in an _____ head injury, and _____ changes may further complicate the condition.

    The neuropathological changes that result from CHI have implications for language and communication. The tendency to characterize language and communication deficits in CHI as _____ or subclinical in nature may not only underplay the true severity of these deficits, but may also lead to the _____ of clients. Certainly, the formal aspects of language, which include _____, morphology, _____ and semantics, may pose minimal difficulty for children with CHI. Even when these aspects are impaired after brain injury, children typically _____ them. However, the ability to use the formal aspects of language to engage in communication with others is not so readily recovered following a brain injury. It is the presence of significant impairments in the communicative uses of language which requires clinicians to pay particular attention to _____ and discourse in their assessment and treatment of children with CHI and other _____ brain injuries.

frontal	closed	syntax	grey	haematoma	subtle
mismanagement		prosody	metabolic	white	recover
occipital	haemorrhages	oedema	intact	phonology	
open	parietal	pragmatics	axonal	traumatic	bony

(4) Which of the following statements is *true* of the language skills of children who sustain a traumatic brain injury (TBI)?
   (a) Children with TBI do not typically differ from normal children on measures of the amount and complexity of sentences in narrative discourse.
   (b) Children with TBI display deficits on tasks of word fluency.
   (c) Children with TBI display intact performance on language tasks that require inferencing.
   (d) Children with TBI display impaired confrontation naming.
   (e) The language deficits of children with TBI are often overlooked and untreated.

(5) Which of the following statements is *false* of discourse in children who sustain a TBI?
   (a) Children with TBI produce fragmented narratives which are difficult to follow.
   (b) Discourse deficits are consistently related to formal language impairments in children with TBI.
   (c) Discourse measures are less sensitive to the communication sequelae of paediatric TBI than classic language measures.
   (d) Narrative discourse has been examined in children with TBI more than other forms of discourse.
   (e) Discourse deficits in children with TBI are more prevalent and persistent than specific language problems.

(6) *True* or *False*: Children with TBI display deficits in written narratives which include the use of incomplete episodic structure.

(7) *True* or *False*: Executive function deficits are among the persistent sequelae of head trauma sustained during childhood.

(8) Children with severe TBI are unable to integrate information across sentences, although they can retain isolated pieces of information. This feature may be related to a failure to generate a _____ representation of the meaning of discourse.

(9) Which of the following discourse problems is explained by poor inhibitory control in children with TBI?
   (a) an inability to grasp the central meaning of discourse
   (b) the intrusion of tangentially related information into discourse
   (c) an inability to conceive of alternative interpretations of a text
   (d) difficulty unfolding discourse in a coherent way
   (e) impairment in the episodic structure of narrative discourse

(10) While structured language assessments capture problems in a proportion of children with TBI, discourse measures are a more sensitive measure of the _____ communicative sequelae in a majority of children with TBI.

3.7   Landau-Kleffner syndrome

(1) In which of the following conditions is language disorder related to the presence of seizures?
  (a) benign rolandic epilepsy
  (b) developmental phonological disorder
  (c) Landau-Kleffner syndrome
  (d) developmental verbal dyspraxia
  (e) developmental dyslexia

(2) Fill in the blank spaces in these paragraphs using the words in the box below:
Landau-Kleffner syndrome (LKS) is a disorder which is not frequently encountered by speech-language pathologists. It was first described in 1957 by Dr William M. _____ and Dr Frank R. Kleffner. Other terms that are used for this disorder include infantile acquired aphasia, acquired epileptic aphasia and aphasia with convulsive disorder. These terms variously reflect the late _____ of the disorder (it is 'acquired' during childhood) and the fact that the aphasia is associated with _____ activity (the aphasia is 'epileptic' or occurs in the presence of a 'convulsive' disorder). Although LKS is a _____ disorder, typically accounting for only 0.2% of all childhood epilepsy, it has a higher _____ in special settings (e.g. _____ for children with severe, specific disorders of speech and language). The disorder is _____ commonly seen in boys than in girls.

Onset of LKS can vary widely from 18 months to 13 years, with a peak incidence between 4 years and 7 years. Loss of language can occur abruptly or _____, with receptive language first to be affected. Expressive deficits usually occur later than receptive deficits and are thus considered to be _____ to the receptive impairment. Children with LKS may no longer recognize spoken words. The verbal _____ is often confused with sudden deafness, although hearing is _____ when assessed. Additional impairments can occur alongside deterioration in language. These include behavioural problems like _____ and aggressiveness as well as _____ deficits. This clinical picture is not present in all cases. Some children with LKS do not display verbal auditory agnosia and _____ has been reported on occasion.

rare	incidence	hyperactivity	prognosis	less
epileptiform	auditory agnosia		impaired	stuttering
residential schools		emotional	onset	prevalence
Landau	cognitive	more	secondary	normal	insidiously

(3) *True* or *False*: There is a relationship between aphasia and abnormal electroencephalogram (EEG) activity in Landau-Kleffner syndrome.

(4) *True* or *False*: Paroxysmal epileptic discharges occur in the perisylvian region of the left hemisphere only during sleep.

(5) Which of the following is *not* a feature of the language impairment in Landau-Kleffner syndrome?
    (a) impaired auditory short-term memory
    (b) impaired phonological processing
    (c) impaired prosodic expression and perception
    (d) impaired reading and writing
    (e) impaired grammatical morphology

(6) The language prognosis in children with Landau-Kleffner syndrome can be highly variable and is dependent on a number of factors. Which of the following factors is influential in determining the long-term language outcome of these children?
    (a) child's age at onset of LKS
    (b) child's executive function skills
    (c) intensity of epileptic activity
    (d) child's motor skills
    (e) duration of LKS

(7) *True* or *False*: Some children with LKS also have non-verbal auditory agnosia, i.e. they are not able to decode non-speech (i.e. environmental) sounds.

(8) *True* or *False*: LKS is considered to be an exceptionally severe form of a common, inherited epileptic syndrome known as benign partial epilepsy with rolandic spikes.

(9) Complete language recovery occurs in all/most/few children who develop LKS (underline <u>one</u>).

(10) Which of the following statements is *true* of the management of children with LKS?
    (a) Signing is used to establish an alternative means of communication.
    (b) Surgical intervention is contraindicated, particularly in children under 7 years.
    (c) Treatment may include the use of anti-epileptic drugs such as valproic acid.
    (d) Surgical intervention may include a procedure called multiple subpial transection.
    (e) Non-verbal communication is not a priority of communication intervention.

Section B: Data analysis exercises

3.8 Developmental phonological disorder 1

Background

The following data are the single-word productions of a 7-year-old Brazilian girl, known as D, who was studied by Yavas and Hernandorena (1991). This girl is a monolingual Portuguese speaker. D displayed normal physical development, has a normal oral mechanism and hearing, and has no neurological problems. According to Yavas and Hernandorena, D displays a systematic sound preference.

	Portuguese	English	Phonemic norm	Client production
1	caixa	box	/káyʃa/	[tátʃa]
2	igreja	church	/igréʒa/	[idéʤa]
3	queixo	chin	/kéʃu/	[tétʃu]
4	acho	I think	/áʃu/	[átʃu]
5	relógio	clock	/ʀelɔʒyu/	[ʀelɔʤu]
6	azulejo	tile	/azúleʒu/	[atúleʤu]
7	bicho	animal	/bíʃu/	[bítʃu]
8	chave	key	/ʃávi/	[tátʃi]
9	chapeu	hat	/ʃapέw/	[tapέw]
10	janela	window	/ʒanέla/	[tanέla]
11	ajuda	help	/aʒúda/	[atúda]
12	marchar	to march	/marʃár/	[matá]
13	achei	I found	/aʃéy/	[atéy]
14	cachorro	dog	/kaʃóʀu/	[tatóʀu]
15	guarda-chuva	umbrella	/guardaʃúva/	[dadatúta]
16	gosto	I like	/gɔstu/	[dɔtu]
17	fogão	oven	/fugãw/	[tudãw]
18	banco	bank	/bãnku/	[bãntu]
19	querido	dear	/kirídu/	[tirídu]
20	aqui	here	/akí/	[atí]
21	guizado	ground beef	/gizádu/	[didádu]

Exercise 1 How are /ʃ/ and /ʒ/ realized by D in the single-word productions in (1) to (7)? What is noteworthy about the context in which these realizations occur?

Exercise 2 Are the realizations of /ʃ/ and /ʒ/, which were identified in response to Exercise 1, maintained in the single-word productions in (8) to (10)? If not, how are these sounds realized in these productions? What is noteworthy about the context of the realizations in (8) to (10)?

Exercise 3 In response to Exercise 1, you may have decided that D is realizing /ʃ/ and /ʒ/ as [ʧ] and [ʤ], respectively, in syllable-initial within word position. Is this pattern of realization maintained in the productions in (11) to (15)? If not, explain how /ʃ/ and /ʒ/ are differently realized in these productions.

Exercise 4 Why do you think /ʃ/ and /ʒ/ are differently realized in (11) to (15)? As a clue to help you, you should examine the context in which these realizations occur. Now try to generate a general rule that captures the realizations of /ʃ/ and /ʒ/ across all the productions in (1) to (15).

Exercise 5 A different type of sound substitution process is present in the single-word productions in (16) to (21). What is the name of this process? This process appears to be entirely separate from the process at work in (1) to (15). One piece of evidence which suggests that this is the case is that where the realizations of /ʃ/ and /ʒ/ did not observe the voicing contrast (i.e. /ʒ/ was realized as [t] on occasion), a voicing contrast is consistently observed in (16) to (21). What other feature of (19) to (21) in particular suggests that the process at work in these single-word productions is quite separate from D's systematic sound preference?

3.8 Developmental phonological disorder 2

Most studies in clinical phonology are conducted in English. This exercise is designed to highlight the much smaller amount of work that has been undertaken into phonological disorder in languages other than English.

Spanish (Puerto Rican dialect)

Background

The following data were obtained from 54 children aged 3;1 to 4;8 years who were identified as phonologically disordered in a study by Goldstein and Iglesias (1996). The sample was comprised of 34 males and 20 females. All children were Spanish–English bilingual speakers who were of Puerto Rican descent. Spanish was the first language of all children and was spoken in the home. These children were enrolled in a Head Start program in Philadelphia, Pennsylvania. Each child passed a pure tone hearing screening bilaterally.

Spanish word	English word	Phonemic norm	Client production
plato	plate	/plato/	[pato]
china	orange	/tʃina/	[ʃina]
plato	plate	/plato/	[pwato]
casa	house	/kasa/	[kaθa]
ratón	mouse	/raton/	[ʀakon]
plate	plate	/plato/	[ato]
dos	two	/dos/	[nos]
jugo	juice	/xuɣo/	[huo]
plato	plate	/plato/	[lato]
tren	train	/tren/	[tlen]
cruce	cross	/krus/	[tlus]
plato	plate	/plato/	[pəlato]
boca	mouth	/boka/	[βoka]
manzana	apple	/mansana/	[pasan]
frio	cold	/frío/	[pío]
cruce	cross	/krus/	[tus]

Italian

Background

Bortolini and Leonard (2000) investigated phonology in 24 Italian-speaking children, 12 of whom had been diagnosed with specific language impairment. The children with SLI, nine girls and three boys, were between 4;1 and 7;0 years of age. In non-language areas, these children were developing normally. Hearing was within normal limits and there was no evidence of neurological impairment. They displayed age-appropriate interactions with objects and other people. Data were elicited by showing the children pictures and asking them to complete sentences. The following productions were of particular interest in this study.

Italian word	English word	Client production
caróta	carrot	[rota]
péttine	comb	[pete]
matíta	pencil	[tita]
martéllo	hammer	[telo]
álbero	tree	[albo]
pécora	sheep	[peka]

Exercise 1 Approximately 93% of the errors produced by the Spanish-speaking children studied by Goldstein and Iglesias fell within a number of commonly occurring phonological processes. These processes included consonant cluster reduction and liquid simplification (i.e. the omission or substitution of any liquid). Provide two examples of each of these processes.

Exercise 2 A number of less commonly occurring phonological processes were also among the 93% of errors committed by these Spanish-speaking children. Velar fronting was one of these processes. Give two examples of this process in the data. This process occurs inconsistently in the data. How would you characterize the contexts in which it does and does not occur?

Exercise 3 Approximately 7% of the Spanish-speaking children's errors fell within a small number of non-targeted phonological processes. These processes included de-affrication, backing and denasalization. Give one example of each type of process in the data.

Exercise 4 The Italian-speaking children with specific language impairment deleted weak syllables in various positions in the word. One such pattern of deletion is word-initial weak syllable deletion. Give three examples of this type of deletion in the above data.

Exercise 5 Among the three productions that you did not include in your answer to Exercise 4 is a different pattern of weak syllable deletion. Does this pattern of deletion affect weak syllables in word-initial, word-medial or word-final position?

3.8 Developmental phonological disorder 3

Background

The following data are the transcribed productions of a girl called Katy who was studied by Pascoe et al. (2005). Katy was 6;5 years at the start of intervention. She comes from a monolingual English home with two parents and an older sibling. Katy has no hearing difficulties and her verbal and performance IQ are 83 and 78, respectively. She is seen by a National Health Service speech and language therapist. Katy attends mainstream school but has a statement of special educational needs. She is a sociable child who enjoys school.

Speech data pre-intervention (6;5 years)

Single-word speech sample

bag	[bæ]	apple	[æ'bə]
web	[wɛ]	garage	['gæwɪ]
fish	[vɪ]	vegetables	['vɛbɛ]
Christmas	[gɪ'mɛ]	sink	[dɪ]
pram	[bæ]	light	[jaɪ]
eggs	[ɛ]	queen	[ki:]
bees	[bɪ]	class	[gæ]

Connected speech sample

Her leg was broken	[ɜ: lɛ: wɒ 'ʔbəuʔə]
A long long time ago	[a lɒ lɒ taɪ 'ʔəgəu]
It's better now	[ɪ 'bɛtə na]
I had playtime already	[ʔaɪ ʔæ 'peɪta i: ʔɔ'wɛdɪ]
It's probably dinner time now	[ɪ 'pwɒ.bɪ 'dɪʔə taɪ na]

Speech data post-intervention (8;2 years)

Single-word speech sample

bag	[bæg]
web	[wɛb]
fish	[vɪ]
Christmas	[gɪ'mɛ]
pram	[pæm]
eggs	[ɛ]
bees	[bɪ]

Connected speech sample

Try on the new shoe for her	[daɪ ɒn dɒ nu: du: fɔ: ʔɜ:]
He be sitting on a lead	[ʔi: bi: 'dɪ.tə ʔɒ ʔa li:d]
He's riding a horse	[ʔi: 'raɪʔɪ a ɔ:t]
He's going over the fence	[ʔɪ 'gɒʔɪ 'ʔɒvə fɛ:]
She fell down the stairs	[dɪ fɔ:n dãu dɛə]

Exercise 1 Katy's pre-intervention speech data reveal a number of phonological processes. Using this data, give <u>two</u> examples of each of the following processes:

(a) prevocalic voicing
(b) deletion of final consonants
(c) deletion of unstressed syllables

Exercise 2 The following productions occur in Katy's pre-intervention speech. Match each production to the correct phonological process:

light [jaɪ]	stopping
queen [ki:]	gliding
sink [dɪ]	consonant cluster reduction

Exercise 3 The following production contains three phonological processes. List these processes: class [gæ]

Exercise 4 On the basis of Katy's post-intervention speech data, which two phonological processes are beginning to resolve in her single-word productions?

Exercise 5 Give two examples of each of the following processes in Katy's post-intervention connected speech:

(a) stopping of fricatives
(b) consonant cluster reduction
(c) vowel distortion

3.9 Specific language impairment 1

Background

Children with expressive specific language impairment (SLI) can display a range of grammatical errors in their spoken output. These errors can affect pronouns, and lexical and auxiliary verbs, amongst other things. Moore (2001) studied 12 children with expressive SLI whose mean age was 4 years and 6 months. Utterances from all 12 children are shown below, alongside their chronological age (year; month).

Age	Spoken utterance
3;11	Her painting.
4;1	Yeah, he sleeping right here.
4;2	He's marrying my dad.
4;2	And her painting now.
4;3	He's a cop.
4;6	She building block.
4;9	Why he fall in the car?
4;10	Then (she's) her eating.
4;10	Her's painting a flower.
5;3	Now, she's washing a glass.
5;4	He kinda has a hat like yours.
5;4	He eating.

Exercise 1 Give <u>one</u> example of each of the following grammatical errors in the above data:

(a) omission of auxiliary verb
(b) use of object pronoun instead of subject pronoun
(c) omission of indefinite article
(d) use of incorrect subject pronoun
(e) immature interrogative form

Exercise 2 Are SLI children of the same chronological age making the same grammatical errors? Present data to support your response.

Exercise 3 Although these children display considerable difficulty in the use of subject and object pronouns, another class of pronouns appears to be less problematic. What is this class of pronouns and give <u>one</u> example of its use?

Exercise 4 Respond with *true* or *false* to each of the following statements:

(a) Noun phrases consistently lack premodifiers in the above data.
(b) These children often omit inflectional suffixes from verbs.
(c) These children only make use of noun phrases and verb phrases.
(d) When auxiliary verbs are used, they agree in number with subject pronouns.
(e) The verb 'is' appears as both an auxiliary and main verb.

Exercise 5 Are more mature grammatical forms consistently found in the older children with SLI? Support your answer with data from the table.

3.9 Specific language impairment 2

Background

Clinical studies of expressive language in children with specific language impairment (SLI) often focus on sentence-level analysis. Less often, extended forms of discourse such as narrative are examined. The following narratives of two boys with SLI were recorded by Bliss et al. (1998). In each extract, 'E' stands for examiner.

Extract 1: Boy with SLI ('R') aged 9;3 years

E: Two weeks ago I had to go to the hospital to have some x-rays taken. Have you ever been to the hospital?

R: Yeah, I had a X-ray because they they're checking on my leg and I was scared that I was going up there and they gave me a balloon and I went to um Toys "Я" Us and gave me a toy but I never . . . . . I uh I just broke my leg and I just fall down on my bike because I got hurt and my Band-Aids on me . . . . put their off and I jumped out of my bike and I . . . I flied and then I jumped down.

E: You jumped down?

R: Uhuh, on the grass . . . . and I um our grandma um she died. She um she was getting older. Our grandma and she died and the uh funeral . . . My ma and dad went to the funeral and then Aunt Cindy was there too and we uh they um uh everybody was sad that um uh that died . . . .and on my birthday I went on my bike and I uh um. . . . I just jump on my bike and I just balance on my . . . . and I did it with uh I did do it with only my hands. I didn't do it without my hands and I uh um one hand too.

Extract 2: Boy with SLI ('L') aged 7;4 years

E: What did you do on vacation?
L: Um . . . . . we went to a ho . . . . . 'n . . . . uh . . . . we went to Sea World and . . . . um . . . . . and um . . . went to the park. We . . . . . we . . . um . . . . . after that . . . it was a long way. We got there to Sea World and the park . . . . and then um . . . . we had a . . . . we . . . um . . . . we went . . . . we . . . . . we . . . . . . we had . . . . . we had drinks the drinks and foot to eat . . . um . . . . we . . . . we had that stuff because I. It was a long way to get there and then . . . . . . um . . . then we um . . . after that we . . . . . It was a short way . . . . . um . . . . It was not a long way to get to the hotel. We went to a hotel . . . . . umm. A girl . . . . 'n.n he, he gave . . . . . . 'n dad gave the keys to . . . . . . to the girl and and then and then and the girl gave the "k," the door keys to the um . . . . to the door . . . and . . . and . . . the door keys to the door then we were in.

Exercise 1 The boy with SLI in extract 1 produces several grammatical errors. Provide <u>one</u> example of each of the following errors:

(a) use of non-finite verb in place of past tense (finite) verb
(b) use of regular past tense -*ed* ending on an irregular verb
(c) incorrect implicit subject pronoun
(d) incorrect preposition in conjunction with an intransitive verb
(e) omission of subject pronoun

Exercise 2 Both boys display problems with referencing with more pronounced difficulties exhibited by the boy in Extract 1. Give <u>one</u> example of each of the following referencing errors:

(a) The use of a subject pronoun without a preceding noun to which it refers.
(b) The use of adverbs which lack a clear referent.
(c) The use of a subject pronoun which has an ambiguous referent.
(d) The use of a definite noun phrase which lacks a preceding referent.
(e) Reverse ordering of indefinite and definite noun phrases of the type that is normally used to introduce new entities into discourse.

Exercise 3 One of these boys displays worse topic management than the other boy. Which boy is this? In what way is his management of topic impaired?

Exercise 4 Narratives can fail if they contain repetitive language. Are there any examples of repetitive language in use in these extracts? Why is repetitive language problematic in narrative discourse?

Exercise 5 Narratives can also fail if they present contradictory or illogical information. Are there any examples of this type of information in the above extracts?

3.9 Specific language impairment 3

Background

The following utterances were produced by a boy known as MM with specific language impairment (SLI) who was studied by Schuele and Dykes (2005). Language samples were collected from this child 12 times between the ages of 3;3 years and 7;10 years. MM was one of four children in a middle-class, Caucasian family with a history of SLI. He was diagnosed with SLI at the age of 3 years by a licensed, certified speech-language pathologist.

Language sample 3 (CA: 3;9 years)

(a) look people doing. Gloss: look what the people are doing.

Language sample 7 (CA: 5;3 years)

(b) they're waiting going somewhere.

Language sample 8 (CA: 5;9 years)

(c) lemme see looks like. Gloss: lemme see what it looks like.
(d) and I don't know that is. Gloss: and I don't know what that is.
(e) it's long ways to go.
(f) let me see he work. Gloss: let me see if he works.

Language sample 9 (CA: 6;2 years)

(g) just watch it goes. Gloss: just watch how it goes.
(h) hmm look that home is. Gloss: hmm look where that home is.
(i) hey, I don't remember has to do. Gloss: hey, I don't remember what it has to do.
(j) this is all the people not got hurt.

Language sample 10 (CA: 6;7 years)

(k) he need catched up.

Language sample 12 (CA: 7;10 years)

(l) I don't know that word is. Gloss: I don't know what that word is.
(m) if you just shoot it and it makes a basket not touching the rim or the the box, it's still a points.
(n) if it if you're walking, if you're bouncing it when you're walking it won't be a foul.
(o) un you look at that picture and you um what are they doing in the picture. Gloss: you look at that picture and you say (or tell) what they are doing in the picture.

Exercise 1 In which of the above utterances do errors occur on WH clauses?

Exercise 2 Examine utterances (b) and (e). What aspect of syntax is in error in (b) but is used correctly in (e)? Is there another utterance in the data in which this same aspect of syntax is impaired?

Exercise 3 What aspect of syntax appears for the first time in the above data in utterances (m) and (n)? Explain how this particular syntactic feature is being used in these utterances.

Exercise 4 How would you characterize the syntactic errors in utterances (f), (j) and (o)?

Exercise 5 What noun phrase errors occur in the above utterances?

3.10 Developmental dyslexia

Background

JR is a 47-year-old right-handed man who has experienced no serious illness, head injury or neurological disorder (Temple 1988). He is self-employed and runs his own building firm. JR's difficulties with reading and spelling started in school and continue to affect his life (e.g. a friend helps him with business paperwork). JR has four children, two of whom also experienced reading and spelling difficulties at school. A third child has autism.

During assessment, JR read 82% of words correctly. Of his errors, 63% were neologisms, 24% were visual paralexias and 12% were morphological paralexias. A visual paralexia occurs when the read word shares at least 50% of the letters in the target word. In a morphological paralexia, the base lexical item of the target word is read correctly but a bound morpheme is dropped, added or substituted. JR's pattern of reading performance can be summarized as relatively good word reading, visual paralexias, morphological paralexias and nonword reading poorer than word reading. This pattern of performance is consistent with a diagnosis of phonological dyslexia.

Data 1: Error types

Target word	Client production
fascinate	fascinated
pivot	pirate
metamorphosis	[mɛtapoɯrʌs]
adventurously	adventurous
systematic	sympathetic
grotesque	[grɔtikə]

Data 2: Non-word reading

Target non-word	Client production
incocidental	incontinental
gracontulation	gran.colt.ulation
cirsemicular	cirsemicircular
compatibinility	compatibility

Data 3: Word reading

Target word	Client production
linguistically	linguistical
belligerently	belly.geenery
existentialism	extentelism
recapitulate	recapulate
prototypical	prototype.on
municipality	Munich . . . muniplayety
presupposition	presumptious
disproportionately	disportionately

Data 4: Irregular word written spelling

Target word	Client written word
cuisine	quizine
kerchief	curchief
meadow	medow
leopard	lepard
friend	freind
honour	honor
jealousy	jelosey
ritual	richual
marriage	marrage
justice	justise
menace	maness
trouble	troble
prairie	prair
health	heath

Data 5: Regular word written spelling

Target word	Client written word
library	libary
effort	efort
victim	victum
fabric	faberic

Exercise 1 The examples in Data 1 exemplify the types of reading errors that JR commits. Provide one example from this table of each of the following types of error:

(a) neologism
(b) morphological paralexia
(c) derivational paralexia
(d) visual paralexia

Exercise 2 In Data 2, JR is attempting to read non-words. What do you notice about the errors he commits? What do these errors tell you about the reading strategy JR is adopting?

Exercise 3 When JR reads short words, he tends to produce visual or morphological paralexias. However, when he reads longer words, as in Data 3, a different type of error occurs. What is this error? What do you notice about each of JR's erroneous productions in this table?

Exercise 4 Respond to each of the following statements about Data 4 with *true* or *false*:

(a) JR's written errors affect only low-frequency words in English.
(b) Errors affect the written spelling of concrete words only.
(c) Written errors affect consonant letters only.
(d) Some written errors involve the omission of one or more letters.
(e) JR's errors violate orthographic rules of English.

Exercise 5 Are JR's written spellings of regular words phonologically valid?

3.11 Intellectual disability 1

Background

The following data have been recorded as part of a longitudinal study of consonant production in a Norwegian girl with cri du chat syndrome. The girl in question, known as Hanna, was studied for nearly five years between the ages of 4;6 and 9;4 years, and is the daughter of the author of the study (Kristoffersen, 2008).

Age	English	Phonemic norm	Client production
4;6	car	/biːl̩/	[pi]
4;6	water	/ʋan/	[mæ]
4;6	ball	/bal/	[pæ]
4;6	crown	/ˈkʰruːnə/	[ˈʉæ]
4;6	draw	/ˈtæjnə/	[ˈhænæ]
4;6	clock	/ˈkʰl̩okə/	[ˈkɔkɔ]
5;9	bucket	/ˈbøtə/	[ˈkatæ]
7;0	battery	/batəˈriː/	[ʋætəˈi]
7;0	key	/ˈnø.kl̩/	[ˈlɔŋ.æ]
7;0	teddy bear	/ˈbamsə/	[ˈpætæ]
9;4	light	/lyːs/	[lyə]
9;4	gnome	/ˈnisə/	[ˈnitæ]
9;4	backpack	/ˈsek/	[ˈtæk]
9;4	roof	/tʰaːk/	[tak]
9;4	flower	/bl̩omst/	[pɔˈlɔt]
9;4	apple	/ˈeplə/	[ˈæpələ]
9;4	snake	/ˈsl̩anə/	[əəˈlaŋæ]
9;4	blue	/ˈbl̩oː/	[pɔˈlɔ]
9;4	bird	/fʉl/	[hul]
9;4	shower	/dʉʂ/	[huə]
9;4	window-the	/ˈʋindʉə/	[ˈʋituə]

Exercise 1 Hanna uses stopping, devoicing and final consonant deletion extensively in her single-word productions. Provide <u>three</u> examples of each of these processes.

Exercise 2 The productions of 'flower', 'apple', 'snake' and 'blue' have a feature in common. As a clue, a sound segment is inserted. What is this segment?

Exercise 3 Describe three instances in the data where a glottal sound replaces an oral sound. Which two sound classes are affected by this substitution?

Exercise 4 Hanna omits various sounds in her productions. Give <u>two</u> examples in the data where nasal and lateral approximant sounds are omitted.

Exercise 5 Use the above data to respond *true* or *false* to the following statements:

(a) Hanna never omits all consonants in her single-word productions.
(b) Hanna cannot achieve the aspiration of plosive sounds.
(c) Hanna displays a sequencing error in her production of 'key'.
(d) Hanna never undertakes a substitution of the alveolar fricative /s/.
(e) The labial approximant /ʋ/ is both a substitution and the target of substitution in Hanna's speech.

3.11 Intellectual disability 2

Background

JB is a boy aged 5;6 years who was studied by McCardle and Wilson (1993). JB has FG syndrome and agenesis of the corpus callosum, the latter confirmed by CAT scan. JB is developmentally delayed. He sat at 15 months, walked at 26 months and used phrases at 3 years. JB had a transient conductive hearing loss between the ages of 2 and 3 years. This was secondary to recurrent otitis media. He displays a friendly, inquisitive personality.

Data

The following conversational exchange between JB and an examiner (E) was recorded during an assessment conducted at 67 months:

E: Tell me about your dog.
JB: It go woof woof.
    I have a doggie, yep.
E: What's your doggie's name?
JB: Spot.
    Spot doggie puppy dog.
    They go pee-pee.
    Go pee-pee (pointing to the floor)
    Smell (holding nose, laughing)

I go fight doggie (kicking the air)
Puppy dog go bite.

Other extracts of JB's expressive language

(1) At 44 months, JB responds as follows when he is asked to stop pushing an equipment cart round the room: 'I wanna push. More push please' (gestures with both hands that he wants one last circuit).

(2) At 54 months, when asked what one should do when tired, JB replied: 'I go sleep uncle room, I sleep uncle bed'.

(3) When asked to name a watch, JB replies: 'Daddy have a pretty'.

(4) When asked to name a match, JB replies: 'fire, burns'.

Exercise 1 In his conversational exchange with the examiner, JB displays a number of grammatical immaturities. One immaturity is a restriction on the number and type of grammatical categories he can use. Using examples, state the grammatical categories to which JB's lexical items belong.

Exercise 2 Is there evidence of morphological immaturity in JB's spoken output? Use data to support your answer.

Exercise 3 A particular feature of the conversational exchange between JB and the examiner suggests that JB's language skills also display lexical immaturity. What is this feature?

Exercise 4 The absence of which <u>four</u> linguistic features confers a telegrammatic quality on JB's utterance in (2)?

Exercise 5 Respond to each of the statements below with *true* or *false*:

(a) JB uses non-verbal communication to augment his poor language skills.
(b) JB's utterances in (3) and (4) are examples of circumlocution.
(c) JB appears to have word-finding problems.
(d) JB's language skills are impaired to the extent that he is not a functional communicator.
(e) JB displays an awareness of pragmatic constraints such as politeness.

3.11 Intellectual disability 3

Background

The following single-word productions were obtained from a sample of 20 children with intellectual disability who were studied by Mackay and Hodson (1982). The children were aged between 6;4 years and 15 years. Among the fifteen males and five females in the sample, there were six children with Down's syndrome. All children passed a hearing screening test.

Target	Client production	Target	Client production
black	[bæ]	toothbrush	[tubwʌ]
ice cubes	[aɪku]	basket	[ægə]
truck	[tⁱʌ]	nose	[noʊ]
gun	[tʌ]	feather	[tɛɚ]
flower	[fa]	television	[tɛəbi]
green	[di]	mouth	[baʊ]
that	[æ] [dæt]	chair	[ʧɛ]
jump rope	[dʌwoʊ]	sled	[ʃɛ]
yo-yo	[moʊjoʊ]	sweater	[sɛɚ]
vase	[bei]	glove	[glʌf]
page	[peiʧ]	music box	[muba]

Background

The phonology of a boy with Down's syndrome was investigated by Bleile (1982). Investigation took place between the ages of 4;0 and 4;7 years. This child's oral structure appeared to be relatively normal apart from a large tongue and a moderate underbite. He also experienced frequent colds and ear infections. This occurred on two occasions during the study. Data was not collected at these times.

Age (year; month)	Target	Client production
4;0	truck	[dəːk]
4;0	farm	[mɑm]
4;0	goat	[dot]
4;0	cheek	[diˑk]
4;0	sheep	[bip]
4;7	cup	[bəːp]
4;7	foot	[duː]
4;7	goat	[dəˑt]
4;7	book	[bɤk]
4;7	duck	[də]
4;7	cheek	[dik]
4;7	dog	[də]
4;7	Ken	[dɛn]

Exercise 1 The children with intellectual disability studied by Mackay and Hodson used a range of immature phonological processes. Five such processes are shown below. Give two examples of each process in the data.

(a) consonant cluster reduction
(b) final consonant deletion
(c) fronting
(d) stopping
(e) postvocalic devoicing

Exercise 2 Several of these children's single-word productions revealed more than one phonological process at work. Indicate these processes in each of the productions below.

(a) ice cubes [aiku]
(b) toothbrush [tubwʌ]
(c) jump rope [dʌwoʊ]
(d) television [tɛəbi]
(e) basket [æɡə]

Exercise 3 Sounds and syllables are frequently deleted by the children studied by Mackay and Hodson. Provide two examples of each of the following deletions in the data.

(a) deletion of word-final syllable
(b) deletion of nasals
(c) deletion of glides
(d) deletion of liquids
(e) deletion of fricatives

Exercise 4 Respond to each of the statements below with *true* or *false*. Each statement relates to the child with Down's syndrome studied by Bleile:

(a) The process of velar fronting resolves during the seven-month period of the study.
(b) The process of stopping resolves during the seven-month period of the study.
(c) At 4;7 years, final consonant deletion is an inconsistent process in this child's speech.
(d) There is evidence of nasal assimilation in this child's speech.
(e) There is evidence of homonymy in this child's phonological system at 4;7 years.

Exercise 5 Among the problematic vowel realizations on display in the speech of this child with Down's syndrome is a failure to use diphthongs. Give two examples of where diphthongs are replaced by monopthongs in the data.

3.11   Intellectual disability 4

Background

The speech of five Dutch-speaking girls with Down's syndrome underwent a phonological process analysis in a study by Van Borsel (1988). The data used in this analysis is shown in the table below. The girls ranged in age from 16;5 years to 19;9 years. The mental ages of these five subjects ranged from 4;4 years to 6;0 years.

Dutch word	English word	Phonemic norm	Client production
plastron	tie	/plasˈtrɔn/	[pasˈtrɔŋ]
trammel	drum	/ˈtrɔməl/	[ˈtumər]
trap	stairs	/trap/	[təˈrap]
trompet	trumpet	/trɔmˈpɛt/	[traˈpɛt]
potlood	pencil	/ˈpɔtloːt/	[ˈpɔtəˈloː]
smurfen	smurf	/ˈsmœrfən/	[ˈsmœfən]
borstal	brush	/ˈbɔrstəl/	[ˈbɔstəl]
olifant	elephant	/ˈoːlifant/	[ˈoːlifan]
hoofd	head	/hoːˈft/	[oːf]
fiets	bike	/fits/	[fit]
muts	cap	/mœts/	[mœs]

Dutch word	English word	Phonemic norm	Client production
zeven	seven	/ˈzeːvən/	[seːvn̩]
ezel	donkey	/ˈeːzəl/	[ˈeːsəl]
kabouter	goblin	/ˌkaˈbɔuter/	[ˌkaˈpultər]
molen	mill	/ˈmoːlən/	[ˈmoːrən]
vlinder	butterfly	/ˈvlɪndər/	[ˈfrɪndə]
ballon	balloon	/baˈlɔn/	[baˈrɔŋ]
tafel	table	/ˈtaːfəl/	[ˈtaːfər]
chocolade	chocolate	/ˌʃoːkoːˈlaːdə/	[soːkəˈlaːdə]
giraf	giraffe	/ʒiˈraf/	[ʐiˈraf]
tafel	table	/ˈtaːfəl/	[taːf]
kabouter	goblin	/ˌkaˈbɔutər/	[ˈbɔutəʳ]
drie	three	/dri/	[kri]
trap	stairs	/trap/	[krap]
citreon	lemon	/siˈtrun/	[siˈkrun]
ballon	balloon	/baˈlɔŋ/	[pəˈrɔŋk]
plastron	tie	/plasˈtrɔn/	[pasˈˈrɔŋk]
telefoon	telephone	/ˌtɪfəˈfɔn/	[ˌtɪləˈfɔŋk]
bril	glasses	/brɪl/	[blɪl]
potlood	pencil	/ˈpɔtloːt/	[ˈpɔploːt]
potlood	pencil	/ˈpɔtloːt/	[ˈpɔkloːt]
trommel	drum	/ˈtrɔməl/	[ˈtlɔŋər]
fiets	bike	/fits/	[fist]
trommel	drum	/ˈtrɔməl/	[ˈtlɔŋər]
piano	piano	/ˌpiˈjaːnoː/	[ˌpiˈjaɲoː]
citroen	lemon	/siˈtrun/	[srun]
tafel	table	/ˈtaːfəl/	[ˈtaːvə]
kabouter	goblin	/ˌkaˈbɔuter/	[ˌkaˈbɔudər]

Exercise 1 Cluster reduction is a feature of the spoken output of these Down's syndrome adolescents. What clusters are reduced in (a) initial position, (b) medial position and (c) final position?

Exercise 2 What phonological processes are evident in the following productions? Give one more example of each process in the data.

(a) vlinder [ˈvlɪndər] → [ˈfrɪndə]
(b) tafel [ˈtaːfəl] → [taːf]
(c) citroen [siˈtrun] → [siˈkrun]

Exercise 3 Two harmony processes are evident in the data: consonant harmony and vowel-consonant harmony, in which the place of articulation of a consonant is influenced by a preceding vowel. Give two examples of each type of harmony process.

Exercise 4 Give two examples of each of the following phonological processes in the data.

(a) devoicing of voiced plosives and fricatives
(b) fronting of palatals
(c) postvocalic voicing

Exercise 5 Some phonological processes occurred only rarely in the spoken output of these adolescents. Four such processes are metathesis, partial reduplication, coalescence and voicing of intervocalic consonants. Which of the following productions represents these processes?

(a) piano [ˌpiˈjaːnoː] → [ˌpiˈjaɲoː]
(b) kabouter [ˌkaˈbɔuter] → [ˌkaˈbɔudər]
(c) citroen [siˈtrun] → [srun]
(d) fiets [fits] → [fist]

3.12 Autism spectrum disorders 1

Background

It is now widely recognized that children and adults with autism spectrum disorder (ASD) experience significant theory of mind (ToM) deficits (Cummings, 2013b, 2014b, 2014c). Theory of mind describes the ability to attribute mental states, such as beliefs, knowledge and intentions, to one's own mind and to the minds of others. ToM deficits result in a number of discourse problems for clients with ASD. Some of these problems are evident in the data below.

Extract 1: Examiner (E) is talking to a 16-year-old boy with autism ('J'), who was studied by Bliss et al. (1998)

E: My sister was on a swing and she fell off and broke her wrist. Have you ever broken your arm?
J: Yeah.
E: What happened?
J: I broke the wrist on his back. I got throat and the stomach and that boy says, 'I got the stomach ache' and the man . . . . and they got . . . . I said, 'I hurt my wrist' and umm the man is umm he's a person. The man is umm he's a and the man is umm . . . . He got arrested and umm the man is got a chest with a body over and the man is uh person of the man of God.

Extract 2: 7-year-old boy with Asperger's syndrome (AS), studied by Loukusa et al. (2007)

The researcher shows the subject with AS a picture of a boy sitting on the branch of a tree, with a wolf underneath the boy at the bottom of the tree. The wolf is growling at the boy. A man with a gun is walking nearby. The researcher reads the following verbal scenario aloud and then asks a question: 'The boy sits up in the tree and a wolf is at the bottom of the tree. How does the boy feel?'

Boy with AS: Fun because he climbs up the tree. I always have fun when I climb up a tree.

Extract 3: 9-year-old boy with Asperger's syndrome (AS), studied by Loukusa et al. (2007)

The researcher shows the boy with AS a picture of a mother and a girl. The girl has a dress on and she is running. There are muddy puddles on the road. The girl has just stepped in the puddle and the picture shows the mud splashing. The researcher reads the following verbal scenario aloud and then asks a question: 'The girl with her best clothes on is running on the dirty road. The mother shouts to the girl: "Remember that you have your best clothes on!" What does the mother mean?'

Boy with AS: You have your best clothes on.

Extract 4: 8-year-old boy with high-functioning autism (HFA), studied by Loukusa et al. (2007)

The researcher shows the boy with HFA a picture of a girl and a boy looking at a video. Their mother comes into the room through the door. The researcher reads the following verbal scenario aloud and then asks a question: 'The children's school starts soon and they should already be on their way to school. However, they are sitting in the nursery looking at a video. Their mother comes to the door and says: "Hurry up!" What does the mother mean?'

Boy with HFA: That he that they should go to the school quickly. Our mother has invented such a clever thing that she has set, set once when I, it-it- is right next to the ki-kitchen the door you go through to the corridor as we live in an apartment building it is there the kitchen door, the clock, is so clever that she has set it she wanted to set it five minutes ahead so that is showed, if it shows like when I must go to the school first on Monday at nine o'clock, must be there nine o'clock sharp, then on Tuesday, on Monday it ends quarter or was it quarter past one or was it one o'clock sharp then on Tuesday I only had a three hour school day . . . (the boy continues in the same vein for several more utterances)

Exercise 1 The boy in Extract 1 introduces a number of referring expressions in the absence of any established referents. This makes his account difficult to follow. Identify <u>four</u> instances where this occurs in his exchange with the examiner. What does this discourse difficulty suggest about this boy's ToM skills?

Exercise 2 The response of the boy in Extract 2 suggests a particular type of ToM difficulty. Which of the following statements best characterizes that difficulty?

  (a) The boy fails to appreciate the knowledge state of the child in the picture.
  (b) The boy believes the man owns the wolf.
  (c) The boy fails to appreciate the emotional state of the child in the picture.
  (d) The boy believes the man is going to hurt the child.
  (e) The boy fails to appreciate the communicative intentions of the child in the picture.

Exercise 3 The boy in Extract 3 merely repeats what the researcher says in his response to the researcher's question. In terms of ToM, explain the boy's error in this case.

Exercise 4 The boy in Extract 4 initially makes an appropriate response to the researcher's question. However, he quickly digresses into an account of events in his own life and the days and times when these occur. Are there any other examples of egocentric discourse in the above extracts? Give an account of egocentric discourse in terms of impaired ToM skills.

Exercise 5 Researchers draw a distinction between cognitive and affective ToM. This is how one group of researchers makes the distinction: 'Cognitive ToM refers to the ability to make inferences about beliefs and motivations, while affective ToM refers to the ability to infer what a person is feeling' (Sebastian et al., 2012: 53). One of the boys in the above extracts displays an affective ToM deficit. Which boy is it?

3.12   Autism spectrum disorders 2

Background

BD is a boy of 8;3 years who was diagnosed as autistic when he first entered school at 4 years (Wolk and Edwards, 1993). The speech-language pathologist at school reported that he had almost no expressive language prior to his seventh birthday. An expressive vocabulary of 50 words was noted at that time. At 7;5 years, BD began to produce two-word utterances. At 8;3 years, he had a productive vocabulary of approximately 400–500 words and his mean length of utterance was 2.0–2.2 morphemes. BD's hearing is normal and he exhibits characteristics which are typical of autism (e.g. withdrawal from social contact and self-abusive behaviour). The use of echolalia and some jargon at the time of data collection led to BD's speech being somewhat unintelligible.

Target	Client production	Target	Client production
spoon	[bu]	snail	[zʌ]
sled	[zʌ]	snake	[zʌ]
glove	[gʌ]	green	[wi]
flag	[w̥ai]	cow	[taω]
sky	[daɪ]	ski	[di]
fruit	[w̥u]	jump	[dʌp]
squirrel	[w̥əʔə]	water	[waʔə]
floor	[w̥aə]	sleeping	[w̥iʔi]
butter	[bʌʔə]	jelly	[dzʌʔi]
tub	[dʌ]	chair	[dzɛə]
truck	[dʌp]	roof	[wu]
rug	[wʌ]	book	[bʌ]
fish	[bet]	leaf	[lip]
thumb	[dʌ]	swing	[w̥in]
spring	[w̥i]	fly	[w̥ai]
late	[leʔ]	horse	[haω]
crayons	[w̥en]	open	[opmʌn]
you	[juju]	by self	[sɛlbaɪ]
three	[w̥i]		

Exercise 1   BD displays a number of immature phonological processes. Five such processes are shown below. Provide <u>two</u> examples of each process in the data:

(a) velar fronting
(b) stopping
(c) final consonant deletion
(d) prevocalic voicing
(e) /s/ cluster reduction

Exercise 2   Several of BD's single-word productions reveal a number of interacting phonological processes. For each production below, indicate the processes which are present:

(a) thumb → [dʌ]
(b) ski → [di]
(c) green → [wi]

Exercise 3   Extensive homonymy in BD's phonological system serves to reduce the intelligibility of his speech. Give <u>three</u> examples of homonymy in the above table.

Exercise 4   There was glottal replacement of intervocalic consonants in many of BD's productions. Give <u>two</u> examples of this process as it affects stops and liquids.

Exercise 5   As well as consonant errors, BD also displayed some unusual vowel changes. Give <u>four</u> examples of these changes in the data.

3.12   Autism spectrum disorders 3

Background

The data below are from a 16-year-old girl called Helen who was studied by Stribling et al. (2007). She has autism and severe learning difficulties. Her verbal interactions with others reveal extensive use of repetition. In the following exchanges, Helen (H) interacts with a number of adults including her mathematics teacher Nigel (N) and her dedicated learning supporter Ginny (G).

Extract 1: Helen and Ginny are making a picture of a mountain

G: now how're we going t'do our mountain
H: (overlaps with) mountain mountain mountain
G: we got t'make it quite big

Extract 2: Helen is taking part in a mathematics class

N: c'n you point to the take away sign
H: (overlaps with) way sign way sign

Extract 3: Helen is taking part in a mathematics class

N: an when you add six an two together
H: eight
N: you get number
H: eight eight eight
N: that's right Helen number eight

Extract 4: Helen requests crisps of Ginny

(Helen is gazing towards a bowl of crisps. She extends her left arm towards the bowl and rotates her hand)

H: crisps crisps crisps
G: (moves plate towards Helen, places plate on table and withdraws arm)
H: crisps crisps
G: (leans forward)
G: you say please

Extract 5: Helen counts blocks

H: one (hands block to N)
H: two (withdraws left hand)

N: (withdraws right hand)
H: (reaches out to left hand block, passes block and places it in Nigel's hand)
H: (simultaneously with above actions) three three three
N: (overlap with Helen's last word) three
N: (lifts right arm and moves right arm forwards)
H: (withdraws left hand)
N: (withdraws right hand)
H: (grasps/lifts left hand block)
H: four
N: four

Exercise 1 Extracts 1 and 2 reveal two types of repetition present in Helen's verbal output. One of these forms of repetition – echolalia – is dependent on a speaker's prior turn. Describe how echolalia is manifested in these extracts.

Exercise 2 The second type of repetition in Extracts 1 and 2 – palilalia – does not involve the repetition of a word just uttered by the previous speaker. Describe how palilalia is manifested in these extracts.

Exercise 3 Repetition assumes a number of functions in Helen's verbal output. What function is performed by Helen's repetition of 'eight' in Extract 3?

Exercise 4 Helen's use of repetition in Extract 4 is quite different from her use of it in Extracts 1 to 3. Describe how Helen is using repetition differently in Extract 4 compared to these earlier extracts.

Exercise 5 In Extract 5, describe how repetition functions in relation to the non-vocal activities in this exchange.

3.13 Childhood traumatic brain injury

Background

The following narrative was produced by a girl with traumatic brain injury, aged 7;4 years, who was studied by Biddle et al. (1996). The girl had no premorbid history of learning or emotional difficulties. She was asked to recount an occasion when she was stung by a bee.

Data

Ummm, I, once, there was a, we went. There was a for. There was this umm fort. A tree fell down. And there was dirt, all kinds of stuff there. It was our fort. And one day, I have a friend named Jude. She's umm grown up. She has a kid. She has a cat named Gus, a kitten. It's so cute. But once, when she didn't have that kitten, one day, me, my brother, my cousin Matt, and her, and my dad, and one of his friends, went into the woods to see the fort, to show her. And we went up there. I stepped on a bee's nest. And they chased us all the way back. And I got stung and my cousin Matt got stung in one of the private parts. And umm I had a bite right here (points), right here (points), right there (points), and umm one on my cheek. And right here. And when I umm went over, when we got back to my friend Jude's house, in her bathroom she had this clean kind of stuff. And I put it on me.

She put it one me right here (points). But umm, I had to go to the bathroom to put it on, you know. It hurt! And my brother Jason he got stung once. He got stung I think three right here (points). I remember where I got stung, but I don't remember where Jason got stung. My friend Jude didn't even get stung. She ran so fast that she didn't even get stung. The bees chased us and I looked back. And there was one right in front of my face. That's when I got stung here (points). There was like two hanging around my legs. I was running and trying to get them off me. They both went, 'Bzzzzz'. It hurt! I was crying my head off.

Exercise 1 A number of discourse problems contribute to this child's difficulty with narrative production. Give <u>one</u> example of each of the following problems in the data:

(a) Utterances are started and then completely abandoned.
(b) Referring expressions lack clear referents.
(c) The narrative digresses into irrelevant detail.
(d) Misuse of temporal expressions which contribute to narrative structure.
(e) Repetitive language which does not advance narrative.

Exercise 2 This child displays reasonably competent use of cohesion in discourse. Give <u>three</u> examples of how she achieves discourse cohesion.

Exercise 3 Respond with *true* or *false* to each of the following statements:

(a) The child uses pointing gestures to compensate for a word-finding difficulty.
(b) The narrative is difficult to follow in parts because of grammatical difficulties.
(c) The child digresses from, but returns to, a particular point or topic.
(d) The child displays some awareness of narrative structure.
(e) The child produces several semantic paraphasic errors in her narrative.

Exercise 4 This child takes her listener's state of knowledge into account as she develops her narrative. Suggest <u>three</u> ways in which she achieves this.

Exercise 5 Which of Grice's maxims appear to be most compromised by the above narrative? Use features of the narrative to support your response.

3.14 Landau-Kleffner syndrome

The following case study concerns a young boy called Dillon who was studied by Alpern (2010). Nearly a year after Dillon first began to display atypical behaviours, he received a diagnosis of Landau-Kleffner syndrome. Examine the details of Dillon's case and then answer the questions below.

Case study: Dillon

Dillon was around 3;5 years of age when his preschool teachers first began to raise concerns with his parents. Prior to that time, Dillon had appeared to be a normally developing, responsive child who had no language delays or evident illnesses. Dillon's teachers reported that he displayed a lack of response in class and that he appeared to 'get lost in the group'. These changes in behaviour had not been detected by Dillon's parents at home. However, when Dillon was observed by them in class, he had poor eye contact and did not play with the other children. Although hearing loss was suspected when Dillon failed to respond when called in class, an audiological assessment revealed no problem with hearing.

At 4;1 years, Dillon was evaluated by his school district. Although he qualified for occupational therapy – his assessment revealed delays in fine motor skills – he achieved high scores on standardized language tests and did not qualify for speech-language services. Nonetheless, Dillon's teachers were still concerned as they did not believe his language test results were consistent with the behaviours they were observing in the classroom.

Nearly a year after teachers first began to raise concerns about Dillon, he experienced a severe regression in language skills. At that point, Dillon was assessed by a neurologist who diagnosed pervasive developmental disorder. Dillon's parents made a video recording of him at 4;4 years. The recording revealed a child who appeared to be in a world of his own. Dillon was unresponsive to his mother and avoided eye contact with her. Despite repeated maternal attempts to engage him in interaction, Dillon appeared to be singing to himself. Although he had some contextually appropriate language, word order was incorrect (e.g. 'I'm pizza eating'). There was also some evidence of confusion, e.g. Dillon said 'I wanna bigger bigger piece' but then pointed to his own piece and said 'This one I want'. At one point in the video, it is clear that Dillon's father believes that he cannot hear him, as he calls Dillon's name with increasing loudness until he responds. In an interaction around a board game with his mother and sister, Dillon displayed some emotional lability. Although he is seen to shout 'I won. I won. Megan lost', he then started to cry because he thought he had lost.

The day after this video recording was made, Dillon was taken to the emergency room where he had a myoclonic seizure. Dillon was placed on valproic acid to control the seizures, but he had a poor response to this medication. After a consultation with a second neurologist, Dillon was admitted to hospital for overnight EEG assessments during a 3–5 day period. Frequent seizures were recorded on the fourth night and Dillon was diagnosed as having Landau-Kleffner syndrome. Intravenous immunoglobulin (IVIG) treatments were chosen over high-dose steroids by his parents as they had concerns about the side effects of the latter medication.

Dillon's communication and other behaviours began to return to pre-illness levels within two weeks of IVIG treatments. However, there were subtle communication difficulties remaining, for which Dillon received speech-language intervention. For example, when retelling a story, Dillon wandered off-topic or focussed on details which were not important. Dillon also failed to elaborate upon his responses, and displayed phonemic paraphasias, word-finding deficits and pronoun confusion. He was also not particularly verbal in a group setting. After the passage of five years, with some of that time spent in either individual or classroom-based speech-language intervention, Dillon had not experienced a relapse in his language skills. Although he is functioning well in a classroom setting, some difficulties with attention, executive function and emotional sensitivity remain.

Exercise 1 Prior to a diagnosis of Landau-Kleffner syndrome, two other conditions were believed to be responsible for Dillon's behaviours. What were those conditions? Explain why these conditions were plausible, even though mistaken, accounts of Dillon's symptoms.

Exercise 2 Dillon's performance on standardized language tests at 4;1 years clearly surpassed his communicative performance in the classroom at around the same time. Explain this difference in terms of the language skills at work in these contexts.

Exercise 3 Which of the following statements characterize Dillon's language skills at 4;4 years during a video-recorded interaction with his mother?

(a) There is a severe deficit of pragmatic language skills.
(b) Dillon's expressive language reveals syntactic deficits.
(c) Receptive language appears to be more impaired than expressive language.
(d) Dillon's expressive language reveals intact grammatical morphology.
(e) Dillon's expressive language reveals pronoun confusion.

Exercise 4 Apart from language, Dillon's cognitive skills have also been compromised by his nocturnal seizures. Which cognitive skills are impaired and is there any evidence that they have an impact on Dillon's use of language?

Exercise 5 Dillon's story-telling abilities after IVIG treatment were clearly problematic and reveal impairment in certain language skills. In which of the following language areas are Dillon's skills impaired?

(a) phonology
(b) semantics
(c) syntax
(d) pragmatics
(e) discourse

SUGGESTIONS FOR FURTHER READING

Benner, G. J. and Nelson, J. R. 2014. 'Emotional disturbance and communication', in L. Cummings (ed.), *Cambridge handbook of communication disorders*, Cambridge: Cambridge University Press, 125–40.

Christo, C. 2014. 'Developmental dyslexia', in L. Cummings (ed.), *Cambridge handbook of communication disorders*, Cambridge: Cambridge University Press, 88–108.

Cummings, L. 2008. *Clinical linguistics*, Edinburgh: Edinburgh University Press (sections 3.2, 3.3, 4.3 and 4.4).

  2014a. *Communication disorders*, Houndmills: Palgrave Macmillan (chapter 3).

De Villiers, J. 2010. 'Autism spectrum disorders', in L. Cummings (ed.) *Routledge pragmatics encyclopedia*, London and New York: Routledge, 31–2.

Ellis Weismer, S. 2014. 'Specific language impairment', in L. Cummings (ed.), *Cambridge handbook of communication disorders*, Cambridge: Cambridge University Press, 73–87.

Norbury, C. F. 2014. 'Autism spectrum disorders and communication', in L. Cummings (ed.), *Cambridge handbook of communication disorders*, Cambridge: Cambridge University Press, 141–57.

Rvachew, S. 2014. 'Developmental phonological disorder', in L. Cummings (ed.), *Cambridge handbook of communication disorders*, Cambridge: Cambridge University Press, 61–72.

Ryder, N. 2010. 'Pragmatic language impairment', in L. Cummings (ed.) *Routledge pragmatics encyclopedia*, London and New York: Routledge, 338–40.

Short-Meyerson, K. and Benson, G. 2014. 'Intellectual disability and communication', in L. Cummings (ed.), *Cambridge handbook of communication disorders*, Cambridge: Cambridge University Press, 109–24.

Chapter 4

Communication disorders in mental illness

Clients with a range of mental illnesses form an increasingly significant part of the caseload of speech and language therapists. Conditions such as schizophrenia have adverse implications for language and communication. Specific linguistic features include a reduction in the amount of spoken output (poverty of speech) and a reduction in the amount of content expressed through speech (poverty of content of speech). Clients with schizophrenia may also make bizarre and irrelevant contributions to a conversational exchange, interpret non-literal and figurative language in a literal way, and fail to observe linguistic politeness in their interactions with others. Alongside marked deficits in pragmatics and discourse, impairments in syntax and semantics are also commonly observed. For example, clients with schizophrenia produce syntactic gaps, e.g. 'he was blamed for and I didn't think that was fair' (Chaika and Alexander, 1986). Clients with bipolar disorder exhibit some of these same linguistic features (e.g. tangentiality). However, they can also display linguistic behaviours which are rarely seen in clients with schizophrenia (e.g. pressured speech).

There is increasing recognition among clinicians and educators of the significant language and communication problems which occur in children with emotional and behavioural disorders. These disorders include attention deficit hyperactivity disorder (ADHD), conduct disorder and selective mutism. The child with ADHD may interrupt others during conversation, blurt out answers before questions have been completed, display frequent topic shifts in conversation, and initiate conversation at inappropriate times. Alongside these pragmatic anomalies, deficits in expressive and receptive language skills have been frequently reported in children with emotional and behavioural disorders (see Cummings 2009, 2014a for discussion).

Section A: Short-answer questions

4.1 Schizophrenia

(1) Fill in the blank spaces in these paragraphs using the words in the box below:
Schizophrenia is a serious _____ that affects approximately one in every hundred people. Although the disorder affects men and women in _____ numbers, its clinical manifestation occurs _____ in men – the late teenage years and early twenties as opposed to early thirties in women. Schizophrenia adversely affects every aspect of an individual's social, occupational and academic functioning. Language and communication are no exception, with deficits in both areas presenting a considerable barrier to the integration of the person with schizophrenia into society.

Clinical studies have examined the language and communication skills of people with schizophrenia in some detail. These studies have revealed deficits in the _____ and syntax of language, while _____ appears to be relatively intact. Inflectional and derivational morphemes are sometimes omitted in spoken output. For example, the person with schizophrenia may say 'help' for *helped* (omission of _____ morpheme) and 'medicate' for *medication* (omission of _____ morpheme). Notable syntactic problems include the use of incomplete phrases, as in 'Do you have?', where the _____ of the verb has been omitted, and incomplete clauses. A client with schizophrenia may open clauses with _____ conjunctions such as *because* and *after* but fail to complete them. Lexical choices are often bizarre and _____ may be evident in spoken output (e.g. use of 'geshinker' in *I got so angry I threw a dish at the geshinker*). The client with schizophrenia can also repeat phrasal elements and nonsense elements in a behaviour known as verbal _____.

A further area of verbal communication that is markedly deviant in schizophrenia is _____ . Clinical studies have shown that speakers with schizophrenia perform poorly on tests of discourse planning/comprehension, understanding humour, sarcasm, metaphors, indirect _____ and the generation/comprehension of emotional prosody. Studies have also found that clients with schizophrenia are unable to recognize when _____ maxims have been violated. This is consistent with the observation that these clients are unable to adhere to these maxims in their own conversational contributions. Lengthy and tangential responses that fail to address a speaker's question or otherwise miss the point of a prior speaker's conversational turn are clear breaches of the _____ and _____ maxims, respectively.

relation	phonology	autism spectrum disorder	equal
coordinating	neologisms	earlier	object
mental illness	subordinating	phonetics	quantity
paraphasia	perseveration	pragmatics	manner
speech acts	personality disorder	derivational	
		conversational	
		morphology	
		inflectional	
		circumlocution	

(2) Which of the following statements characterize schizophrenia in adults?
   (a) Schizophrenia is diagnosed on the basis of negative and positive symptoms.
   (b) To date, there is no evidence of a genetic basis to the disorder.
   (c) Most clients with schizophrenia make a complete recovery within five years of a first psychotic episode.
   (d) Auditory hallucinations are believed to be responsible for the pragmatic disturbances in schizophrenia.
   (e) Pragmatic impairments in schizophrenia have been linked to cognitive deficits.

(3) *True* or *False*: The aetiological basis of schizophrenia has not yet been conclusively established.

(4) *True* or *False*: Glossomania is a feature of schizophrenia in which morphological associations are developed during long sequences of utterances.

(5) *True* or *False*: The relationship of thought disorder to language performance in schizophrenia is unclear.

(6) Which of the following is *not* a linguistic or communication feature of schizophrenia?
   (a) neologisms
   (b) phonemic paraphasias
   (c) perseveration
   (d) lexical retrieval problems
   (e) glossomania

(7) Which of the following is an expressive pragmatic deficit in schizophrenia?
   (a) difficulty recovering the implicatures of utterances
   (b) difficulty establishing the illocutionary force of speech acts
   (c) difficulty contributing to conversation utterances which adhere to Gricean maxims
   (d) difficulty comprehending metaphors and idioms
   (e) difficulty producing utterances which contain embedded clauses

(8) Diagnostic criteria for schizophrenia are contained in the _____ which is published by the American Psychiatric Association.

(9) A diagnosis of schizophrenia is based on the presence of positive and negative symptoms. The positive symptoms of the disorder include thought disorder, _____ and hallucinations. Negative symptoms of schizophrenia include affective flattening, _____, apathy, avolition and social withdrawal.

(10) Discourse deficits in schizophrenia include problems with _____ and coherence.

4.2 Bipolar disorder

(1) Bipolar disorder is a psychiatric disorder in which the patient's mood alters between _____ episodes, depressive episodes and episodes of _____ mood.

(2) The depressed speaker may exhibit _____ retardation in slowed speech and thinking.

(3) *True* or *False*: Flight of ideas in mania is essentially indistinguishable from derailments in schizophrenia.

(4) Which of the following is *not* a feature of communication in the depressed speaker?
   (a) reduction in the amount of talk
   (b) reduced variety of the content of talk
   (c) extensive use of circumlocution
   (d) reduced variation in intonation
   (e) negative words (e.g. not, never) tend to predominate in the verbal output

(5) Which of the following are communication features of manic episodes in bipolar disorder?
   (a) poverty of speech
   (b) high rates of initiating exchanges across contexts and topics
   (c) pressured delivery of speech
   (d) theatrical speech
   (e) agrammatism

(6) Fill in the blank spaces in these paragraphs using the words in the box below:
People with bipolar disorder experience marked mood swings which range from depression through to _____. These affective states are the basis of the older term which was used to describe this disorder, _____. Although these affective states are afforded most attention, in reality they lie on a continuum with other states in between them. One of these states is _____, a form of remission in which there is normal emotional regulation. Another state is _____, during which an individual can sometimes experience creativity and enhanced performance in certain domains. Not all these states are experienced by individuals who have bipolar disorder. Individuals

with Bipolar I experience the full range of states from ———— to hypomania and on to mania. However, individuals with Bipolar II only experience depression and hypomania, but not full-blown ————. Between these states, periods of ———— can last for years or, in some cases, hours.

Individuals with bipolar disorder can display some of the same linguistic behaviours that are seen in schizophrenia. For example, there is ———— in both conditions, with the speaker displaying an inability to sustain goal-directed conversation. There is also disregard for conversational conventions in both disorders. However, the speaker with bipolar disorder can also display linguistic behaviours that are rarely seen in schizophrenia. Two such behaviours are pressured speech and flight of ideas. In pressured speech, excessive speech is produced at a ———— rate which it is difficult to interrupt. It is one of the hallmarks of ———— and manic speech. The speaker with mania who is experiencing flight of ideas engages in frequent ———— shifts during conversational narratives. These shifts are accompanied by ———— speech and can often include wordplay.

topical	remission	circumstantiality	depression
psychotic disorder	rapid	hypomania	tangentiality
mania	erratic	manic-depressive illness	glossomania
euthymia	hypomanic	pragmatic	pressured

(7) *True* or *False*: Poverty of speech is not a feature of language in bipolar disorder.

(8) *True* or *False*: The male:female sex ratio in bipolar disorder is approximately 10:1.

(9) *True* or *False*: Illogicality is a feature of language in bipolar disorder.

(10) During clang associations, the speaker with bipolar disorder produces strings of words that are similar in ———— and often rhyme.

4.3 Emotional and behavioural disorders

(1) Which of the following is *not* an emotional and behavioural disorder in children?
   (a) conduct disorder
   (b) selective mutism
   (c) Tourette's syndrome
   (d) attention deficit hyperactivity disorder
   (e) oppositional defiant disorder

(2) Which of the following are communication features of attention deficit hyperactivity disorder (ADHD) in children?
   (a) The child with ADHD does not listen when spoken to directly.
   (b) The child with ADHD often talks excessively.
   (c) The child with ADHD blurts out answers before questions have been completed.
   (d) The child with ADHD commences conversational turns at appropriate junctures.
   (e) The child with ADHD produces jargon in spoken output.

(3) *True or False*: For a diagnosis of selective mutism to be made, a child must demonstrate a consistent failure to speak in all contexts and settings.

(4) *True or False*: Social anxiety is frequently found in children with selective mutism.

(5) *True or False*: There is evidence of pragmatic impairment in children with conduct disorder.

(6) *True or False*: Some investigators argue that reading problems may contribute to the early onset of conduct disorder.

(7) Fill in the blank spaces in this paragraph using the words in the box below:

Pragmatic language skills in children with emotional and _____ disorders have received relatively little attention in the clinical literature. This is despite the fact that conversational behaviours are included among the diagnostic features of at least one of these disorders in the _____ (DSM). Inattention, _____ and _____ in attention deficit hyperactivity disorder (ADHD) are associated with several conversational problems. According to DSM, the individual with _____ displays frequent shifts in conversation, does not listen to others and does not keep his or her mind on conversations. Hyperactivity may be expressed by _____ talking. The impulsive individual may blurt out _____ before questions have been completed, may make comments out of turn, fail to _____ to directions, initiate conversations at inappropriate times and _____ others excessively. These various conversational behaviours have a negative impact on the _____ skills of the child with ADHD and, as such, are targets of intervention.

social communication	psychological	listen	excessive
impulsivity	unintelligible	behavioural	theory of mind
Diagnostic and Statistical Manual of Mental Disorders		interrupt	
hyperactivity	utterances	answers	inattention

(8) Which of the following is *not* associated with selective mutism in children?
   (a) There are often delays in motor and cognitive development.
   (b) The failure to communicate is on account of language impairments.
   (c) Auditory comprehension skills are generally within the normal range.
   (d) The failure to communicate is on account of speech impairments.
   (e) Selective mutism has adverse implications for social communication.

(9) Which of the following statements characterizes the prevalence of conduct disorder?
   (a) Conduct disorder is more common in girls than in boys.
   (b) Conduct disorder is more common in boys than in girls.
   (c) Conduct disorder has a similar prevalence in boys and girls.
   (d) There is a higher prevalence of conduct disorder in individuals with genetic syndromes than in the general population.
   (e) There is a higher prevalence of conduct disorder in incarcerated individuals than in the general population.

(10) Defiant and noncompliant behaviours are types of internalizing/externalizing problems (underline one).

Section B: Data analysis exercises

4.4 Schizophrenia 1

Background

The spoken language of adults with schizophrenia is characterized by a range of anomalies. One such anomaly is verbal perseveration. During verbal perseveration, schizophrenic clients continue to use a linguistic form beyond the point where it is appropriate to do so. The perseverated form can be used in the client's next utterance (e.g. 25 and 26 in the table below) or after several intervening utterances (e.g. 18 and 39 in the table below). Barr et al. (1989) argue that verbal perseverative errors are related to executive dysfunction in schizophrenia. These investigators assessed the confrontation naming performance of 15 subjects (8 male, 7 female) with chronic schizophrenia. The mean duration of these patients' psychiatric illness was 10;9 years. All subjects, who ranged in age from 25 to 46 years, were taking neuroleptic medication at the time of the study.

Item	Stimulus	Client response
35	harmonica	'candy bar ... (stimulus cue) ... harmonica'
38	baby rattle	'bubble ... harmonica ... (phonemic cue) ... rattle'
40	telescope	'microscope, harmonica, molasses ... telescope'
44	harp	'harmonica ... (phonemic cue) ... harticle'
18	octopus	'octopus'
39	cactus	'octatoos ... no, octopus ... no ... the thing you find in Mexico ... (phonemic cue) ... captus'
65	maze	'abstract ... (phonemic cue) ... (no response)'
79	abacus	'math beads, math scale ... (phonemic cue) ... abstract'
25	raft	'raft'
26	wreath	'Christman rath ... no, wreath'
66	nozzle	'nozzle'
71	noose	'noosle ... no, rope ... a noose'

Exercise 1 The perseverated items in some of the clients' responses take the form of blends in which sounds from the repeated word and the target word are brought together. Identify <u>four</u> instances where this occurs in the data.

Exercise 2 Some responses reveal the use of circumlocution before the client is or is not able to produce the target word. Identify <u>two</u> instances where this occurs in the data.

Exercise 3 On at least one occasion, the client's response shares sound and functional features of the target item. Identify this response in the data. Also, two responses reveal a visual relationship between the uttered word and target. Which responses are these?

Exercise 4 Are phonemic cues effective in eliciting target words from these clients?

Exercise 5 A number of the clients' responses involve the use of words which are semantically related to the target form. Give <u>three</u> examples of this type of error in the data.

4.4 Schizophrenia 2

Background

The spoken discourse of adults with schizophrenia can appear anomalous for a range of reasons. On some occasions, the sense of anomaly derives from problems with lexical cohesion. This may occur because the client with schizophrenia is not making correct use of anaphoric reference such as when the pronoun 'she' is used to refer to the dress in the utterances 'Mary bought a dress. She was the pink one'. On other occasions, spoken discourse may display appropriate use of lexical cohesion but can still appear anomalous for other reasons, such as when the client uses cohesive devices to introduce irrelevant points and topics.

The extract below is taken from a study by Chaika and Lambe (1989) of narrative production in 22 psychotic clients. Of these clients, 14 received a discharge diagnosis of schizophrenia and 8 received a diagnosis of mania. The extract was produced by a single schizophrenic client, known as A, following a viewing of a short video story called the Ice Cream Story. In this story, a young girl is refused her request for ice cream from her mother because it is close to supper time. However, when her father enters the house, the young girl approaches him with the same request and he gives her money from his trouser pocket. The young girl takes the money to the store and uses it to buy a very large double-decker cone.

Extract

I was watching a film of a little girl and um s bring back memories of things that happened to uh people around me that affected me during the time when I was living in that area and she just went to the store for a candy bar and by the time ooh of course her brother who was supposed to be watching wasn't paying much attention he was blamed for and I didn't think that was fair the way the way they did that either, so that's why I'm kinda like asking could we just get together for one big party or something ezz it hey if it we'd all in which is in not they've been here, so why you jis now discovering it?

Exercise 1 Does this extract reveal any appreciation of narrative structure on the part of this schizophrenic client?

Exercise 2 Give <u>two</u> examples of where this client is using lexical cohesion appropriately in the extract.

Exercise 3 This client's narrative is highly egocentric in places. Give <u>one</u> example of where such egocentricity occurs.

Exercise 4 During egocentric discourse, it is particularly difficult to follow this client's narrative. Explain why this is the case in terms of the client's use of referential devices.

Exercise 5 Even when this client's discourse is egocentric, it still displays cohesion. Give <u>one</u> example of where these cohesive links occur.

4.4   Schizophrenia 3

Background

Below is an extract of expressive language produced by an adult with schizophrenia who was studied by Chaika (1982). There are a number of linguistic anomalies which make this client's verbal output difficult to follow. Use the following questions to help you characterize the specific linguistic problems which are responsible for the aberrant nature of this client's verbal output.

Data

. . . you should be able to with your thought process your mental process and your brain wave you should be able to acquire the memory knowledge necessary as to study the bible to speak and think in a lord tongue you should be able to memory all the knowledge down on down on the page in the bible book to work for god in the mission now in the position I am in now with the medicate and with the hospital program. I am being helped but at the same time that I am being help with the food and medicate the food and medicate and the the food an medicate and the an the ah rest I feel that I still do not have this I still not have the thought pattern and the mental process and the brain wave necessary to open up a page open up the old testament and start to memory it the old te- the old new testament page of the bible start to have me- memory knowledge ne-cessary to speak to think in the lo- speak and think in the lord's tongue.

Exercise 1 Is there evidence of problems with morphology in this client's spoken output? If so, what morphological errors occur? Is there another way of viewing these difficulties which does not involve their characterization as morphological errors?

Exercise 2 Does linguistic perseveration occur in this client's verbal output? Use data from the extract to support your answer.

Exercise 3 This client is able to reference the topic of his verbal output – his cognitive difficulties with processing written language – through the repeated use of a number of compound nouns. What nouns are performing this role in this extract?

Exercise 4 There is evidence of intact and impaired use of verbs in this extract. Give <u>two</u> examples of each type of verb use.

Exercise 5 What linguistic features of this extract may indicate that this client is experiencing word-finding difficulties?

4.4   Schizophrenia 4

Background

A 53-year-old male patient with schizophrenia, known as PQ, received speech and language therapy (SLT) for severe poverty of speech (Clegg et al., 2007). PQ had a long history with psychiatric services since he first presented to them at the age of 17 years. His current admission had been preceded by a two-year period in which he experienced severe psychotic and affective symptoms. He reported the following positive and negative symptoms: thought interference (e.g. he believed other people were inserting and removing thoughts from his head), delusional perceptions (e.g. he believed he had sold his soul to the devil when he found a cigarette in what he thought was an empty packet), delusions of reference (e.g. PQ thought the television and radio were communicating with him directly), and negative cognitions (e.g. extreme feelings of guilt). PQ was diagnosed as having para-noid schizophrenia with a concurrent depressive episode. Prior to intervention, PQ had a negative attitude to communication, low self-esteem and high social anxiety. Although his negative attitude to communication remained unchanged following intervention, his self-evaluative status did improve.

Before SLT intervention

Interview between PQ and doctor (DR) during a weekly ward round. The interaction takes 90 seconds in total. PQ's mean length of utterance is 3.4 and the doctor's MLU is 9.4.

DR: Hello PQ, please come in and sit down. Do you know everyone here?
PQ: (Nods his head to indicate yes.)
DR: So how have you been getting on this week?
PQ: Okay (pause of 4 seconds).
DR: I gather the medication has been causing excess salivation, has it been happening a lot?
PQ: Bit of salivation occasionally (pause of 6 seconds).
DR: When does this happen?
PQ: Possibly at night (pause of 8 seconds).
DR: What have you enjoyed doing this week on the ward PQ?
PQ: Possibly relaxation (pause of 2 seconds).
DR: What do you feel you benefit from by doing the relaxation sessions?
PQ: To relax, get a bit uptight (pause of 5 seconds).
DR: Do you feel uptight all the time?
PQ: Occasionally (pause of 3 seconds).
DR: Do you feel less anxious now than when you first came?
PQ: About the same (pause of 3 seconds).
DR: Can you tell me a bit more? Are you feeling less anxious than you were?
PQ: Could be a bit better . . . (pause of 3 seconds) slightly . . . (pause of 4 seconds) possibly.
DR: Does the anxiety affect you all the time?
PQ: Alright on occasions, slightly alright (pause of 8 seconds).
DR: Have there ever been times when you haven't felt very anxious?
PQ: Sometimes, a long time ago (pause of 7 seconds).
DR: Right, okay (pause of 4 seconds) Do you think you're getting better?
PQ: I think I've improved, yes.
DR: In what way?
PQ: Right (pause of 5 seconds).
DR: Is there anything you want to discuss or anything you're worried about.
PQ: Not particularly worried (pause of 8 seconds).
DR: Okay, we'll leave it there, thank you.
PQ: Thank you.

After SLT intervention

Interview between PQ and doctor (DR) during a weekly ward round. The interaction takes 90 seconds in total. PQ's mean length of utterance is 8.5 and the doctor's MLU is 9.5.

DR: Hello PQ, come on in and have a seat.

PQ: Okay, thank you, hello.

DR: You had some leave this week, how did it go?

PQ: Better than I thought (pause of 3 seconds).

DR: Where did you go?

PQ: Went to X (name of location) to stay with my sister Mary.

DR: When did you go?

PQ: My sister Sally, she and her husband took me down in the car and brought me back last week.

DR: What did you do there?

PQ: Went out for a walk, went out for some visits, did some reading in the garden, did a lot of reading actually (pause of 2 seconds).

DR: Okay, are you happy for the plans for the discharge next week?

PQ: Yes (pause of 2 seconds).

DR: Is Tuesday going to be better than the Monday?

PQ: Why Tuesday? Why has it changed?

DR: Oh your brother rang this morning, no one's going to be around on the Monday to collect you so he suggested Tuesday instead.

PQ: Right, okay (pause of 3 seconds).

DR: And you're carrying on seeing X (name of SLT).

PQ: Yes, I'm seeing her this Thursday aren't I (looks at SLT).

DR: Yes, same arrangements as usual, is that still okay?

PQ: Yes fine (pause of 3 seconds).

DR: And what's happening with X (name of day centre)?

PQ: I'm going to do three days no I forgot two or three, I need to check this with X (name of day centre).

DR: When are you seeing X (name of Community Psychiatric Nurse)?

PQ: Tomorrow but she's gradually scaling off she's got a new job so there'll be a new person coming.

DR: Okay and what about the medication, you'll need to go to X (name of hospital) to have your blood checks done.

PQ: Do I just walk in?

DR: You'll be sent an appointment card telling you where to go and when so don't worry you'll be told what to do.

PQ: How often do I go?

DR: It'll be every two weeks.

Exercise 1 The frequency and duration of pauses are considerably less in the post-intervention interview than in the pre-intervention interview. What function are these pauses performing in the pre-intervention interview? Why do they decrease so dramatically in the post-intervention interview?

Exercise 2 In the pre-intervention interview, certain linguistic features are infrequently used by PQ. List these features and suggest why they are infrequently used. What linguistic features are particularly common in the pre-intervention interview?

Exercise 3 The post-intervention interview contains several linguistic features that were not present in the pre-intervention interview. What are these features? Suggest why they emerge post-intervention.

Exercise 4 The use of questions differs in these two interviews. Describe what these differences are and suggest why they might occur.

Exercise 5 PQ's management of topic differs markedly between the pre-intervention and post-intervention interviews. Describe these differences.

4.5 Bipolar disorder

Background

Bipolar disorder (formerly called 'manic depression') is a psychiatric disorder in which the patient's mood alters between manic episodes, depressive episodes and episodes of normal mood known as euthymia. During manic episodes, a patient can exhibit euphoria, restlessness, poor judgement and risk-taking behaviour. During depressive episodes, a patient can display depression, anxiety and hopelessness. It is now widely acknowledged that this psychiatric disorder has adverse implications for language and communication. Some of these implications will be examined in the following data taken from Fine (2006).

Data 1: Exchange between an interviewer (I) and a depressed speaker (S), taken from Fine (2006: 240)

I: Was she willing to take care of the baby?
S: I wouldn't let her . . . no . . . you know . . . I just didn't feel like that um if I couldn't take care of
     her. I didn't want anybody else to
I: Right
S: Plus I didn't want to run into her . . . if I saw her I would keep her
I: Right
S: I don't know . . . I don't know why she turned against me to tell you the truth . . . in fact that's one
     of the reasons . . . she doesn't like A (name), my husband

Data 2: Exchange between an interviewer (I) and a depressed speaker (S), taken from Fine (2006: 245)

I: So we were talking about you and your present condition and that kind of thing
S: Right
I: Is there any way you are . . . all the time would you say I mean that's worse now and . . . other
     things are going on but would you say that by-and-large you always were a rather
     self-conscious person
S: . . . yes I am
I: Do you know where it comes from . . . do you think that as a child you had experiences that made
     you ah . . . become self-conscious and kind of ashamed of some things about yourself
S: . . . hmm . . . it could be

Data 3: Verbal output of a depressed speaker, taken from Fine (2006: 248)

I looked at my bosses . . . I looked at . . . people I could talk to you know people that seem
friendly . . . you know . . . for a little bit of guidance well . . . at the time it didn't work out too
well . . . you know . . . I would take their advice and sometimes it would backfire you know so . . .

Data 4

The following extract of discourse was produced by a manic patient during a videotaped conversation with his psychiatrist. It was recorded by Neale et al. (1984) who are cited in

Goss (2006). The transcription notation used by Goss has been removed. The manic patient had already dominated the conversation for over five minutes at the point at which this extract begins. After glancing down at his yellow shirt, the patient states:

. . . it reminds me of Baba Ramdas or those Tao people ya know singing ha ray ha ray ohm ohm mo (laughs) ya know om backwards is the abbreviation for Missouri and the omni this bar in town is O M N I and backwards I N when I came to St. L or when I came to Indiana in uh seventy six they dropped the D off the I N so omni backwards is I N M O in mo the two states of the universe (laughs) . . .

Exercise 1 Several language features characterize the spoken output of the depressed speaker. Two such features are a reduction in the amount of speech (poverty of speech) and a reduction in the variety of the content of speech (poverty of content of speech). Is either of these features evident in the extracts presented above? Use data to support your answer.

Exercise 2 The speaker with depression often reveals his depressed mood through the excessive use of negative utterances. Which of the above extracts contains an example of this linguistic behaviour? Give three examples of how this behaviour is manifested by the speaker you have identified.

Exercise 3 A depressed speaker often attempts to distance himself from the truth of claims and can seek excessive reassurance from his listener. How are these behaviours manifested by the speaker in Data 3?

Exercise 4 Is the verbal output of the manic patient in Data 4 triggered by a visual stimulus? Provide evidence to support your answer.

Exercise 5 In Data 4, the manic patient's verbal output reveals a complex interplay between sound sequences, letter configurations and semantic associations. Using data from the extract, describe the form that this interplay takes.

4.6 Emotional and behavioural disorders

Background

Attention deficit hyperactivity disorder (ADHD) has significant implications for the communication skills of affected children. These children tend to interrupt other speakers' turns in conversation, do not listen to and follow instructions, and talk excessively. Alongside the behavioural problems of these children, communication impairments can have an adverse effect on academic performance and other domains.

The following conversations between a teacher and two children with ADHD exemplify some of the communication problems of these children. The two children in question, Abraham and Adam, were popular with teachers and their peer groups. The conversations were recorded in primary school special education classes as part of a study by Peets (2009) of classroom discourse in children with language impairment. Transcription notation has been removed and other modifications have been made.

Data 1: Conversation between teacher (T) and Abraham (A) in the presence of students (S)

A: Then I throw the ball at my baby brother.
T: Oh why did you do that?
A: So so he can play with it.
T: Did he like you throwing the ball at him?
A: Yeah because I because when I sometimes throw the ball at him he laughs.
T: So you you just threw it gently.
A: Then then he took the pillow.
S: (unspecified turn)
A: Then I said 'look out' then I then he throw the pillow in my face!
(Students laugh)

Data 2: Conversation between teacher (T) and Adam (A)

A: I went to my cousin's house and when I went to my cousin's house that was later when I when I we went back home for um from snow tubing.
T: Can you tell us about snow tubing?
A: Snow tubing is is freaky.
T: Freaky. Tell us what it's like. What do you do?
A: They uh they have a machine that will they have a hooks that will pull you back up and then you have eight tickets you give one of them to (th)em then you got hold onto a rope they have like a little round thing and then you go they put the put the hook inside and then and then it pulls you back up and then you slide down they put they maybe the if you want to stay straight you tell my parents from up there if you want a spin they he spins you.

Exercise 1 Both Abraham and Adam meet criteria for language impairment. Using data in the above conversations, and the expressive language of Abraham below, give five examples of grammatical deficits in these children.

Abraham: Summer summer is my bestest month because you know why Wonderland and swimming!

Exercise 2 Respond with *true* or *false* to each of the following statements:

(a) Abraham and Adam display an impairment of auditory language comprehension.
(b) Abraham and Adam display appropriate turn-taking skills.
(c) Abraham and Adam produce turns of an appropriate length.
(d) Abraham makes inappropriate use of humour in his exchange with the teacher.
(e) Adam produces some repetitive language in his exchange with the teacher.

Exercise 3 Adam produces an extended turn in his exchange with the teacher. This turn is difficult to follow in parts. Using data to support your answer, explain why this is the case.

Exercise 4 What linguistic expression(s) do both Abraham and Adam use to continue talking in their exchanges with the teacher? What conversational function is this expression performing for these children, particularly Adam?

Exercise 5 Notwithstanding their conversational difficulties, both Abraham and Adam are popular children who are engaging to teachers and their peers. What features of their conversational performance make them desirable interlocutors for others?

SUGGESTIONS FOR FURTHER READING

Bryan, K. 2014. 'Psychiatric disorders and communication', in L. Cummings (ed.), *Cambridge handbook of communication disorders*, Cambridge: Cambridge University Press, 300–17.

Covington, M. A., He, C., Brown, C., Naçi, L., McClain, J. T., Fjordbak, B. S., Semple, J. and Brown, J. 2005. 'Schizophrenia and the structure of language: The linguist's view', *Schizophrenia Research* **77**:1, 85–98.

Cummings, L. 2008. *Clinical linguistics*, Edinburgh: Edinburgh University Press (section 5.6).
    2014a. *Communication disorders*, Houndmills: Palgrave Macmillan (chapter 6).

Fine, J. 2006. *Language in psychiatry: a handbook of clinical practice*, London: Equinox Publishing (chapters 4 to 9 inclusive).

France, J. and Kramer, S. (eds.) 2001. *Communication and mental illness: theoretical and practical approaches*, London and Philadelphia: Jessica Kingsley Publishers (chapters 1, 3, 4 and 6).

Kuperberg, G. R. and Caplan, D. 2003. 'Language dysfunction in schizophrenia', in R. B. Schiffer, S. M. Rao and S. M. Fogel (eds.), *Neuropsychiatry*, second edition, Philadelphia: Lippincott, Williams & Wilkins, 444–66.

Meilijson, S. 2010. 'Schizophrenic language', in L. Cummings (ed.), *Routledge pragmatics encyclopedia*, London and New York: Routledge, 414–16.

Ribeiro, B. T. and De Souza Pinto, D. 2010. 'Psychotic discourse', in L. Cummings (ed.) *Routledge pragmatics encyclopedia*, London and New York: Routledge, 370–4.

Westby, C. and Watson, S. 2013. 'ADHD and communication disorders', in J. S. Damico, N. Müller and M. J. Ball (eds.), *The handbook of language and speech disorders*, Oxford: Wiley-Blackwell, 529–55.

Chapter 5

Acquired speech disorders

Speech disorders can also have their onset in adulthood. Carcinomas of the oral cavity can often be advanced at the point of diagnosis and necessitate surgical removal of the tongue in either a partial or a complete glossectomy. Post-operative speech production can achieve acceptable levels of intelligibility. This is possible through the use of compensatory strategies, which are either naturally acquired or directly taught. These strategies permit the client who undergoes a glossectomy to produce articulatory contrasts in the absence of normal tongue structure and mobility. As with many clients with acquired speech disorders, the individual who has a glossectomy may also present with swallowing problems (dysphagia).

A range of neurological events and diseases can cause acquired dysarthria in adults. Most commonly, this speech disorder is the result of a cerebrovascular accident or stroke. However, several other conditions including infections (e.g. meningitis), traumatic brain injury, brain tumours, and neurodegenerative diseases (e.g. multiple sclerosis) may also give rise to dysarthria in adults. Depending on medical aetiology, acquired dysarthrias may improve, deteriorate or remain stable over time. For example, the adult who sustains a head trauma may be severely dysarthric or anarthric in the period immediately post-injury. But as spontaneous recovery occurs, there may also be improvement in speech function. However, in the client with a progressive neurodegenerative condition like motor neurone disease, speech production will deteriorate over a period of weeks or months as the client's neurological status worsens. These differing patterns of recovery and deterioration demand continual assessment of a client's speech production abilities and rapid adjustments in treatment.

Alongside acquired dysarthria, a client may also present with apraxia of speech. Unlike developmental verbal dyspraxia, there is a clear neurological aetiology of apraxia of speech, most typically a brain lesion caused by a cerebrovascular accident. The co-occurrence of acquired dysarthria and apraxia of speech in clients has resulted in the development of criteria for use in a differential diagnosis of these disorders. Certainly, the significant differences in these motor speech disorders demand quite different assessments and therapies.

Section A: Short-answer questions

5.1 Glossectomy

(1) The most common type of tongue cancer is a _____ carcinoma.

(2) Following glossectomy, a speaker can achieve relatively good intelligibility through the use of adaptations or _____ involving the lips, mandible and pharynx.

(3) Which of the following is *not* a feature of speech in a glossectomy patient?
   (a) Hypernasality which is related to velopharyngeal incompetence.
   (b) The jaw and lips may participate in compensatory articulation.
   (c) Plosive sounds involving the tongue may be substituted by fricatives, glottal stops or bilabial stops.

(d) The epiglottis may be active during the production of speech sounds.

(e) Mobility of remaining tongue tissue is a significant factor in speech intelligibility.

(4) Researchers have been able to draw conclusions about the type of tongue structure after glossectomy which leads to the best speech outcomes. One of their findings is that post-operative lingual _____ is more important to speech acceptability than the _____ of tongue mass remaining after surgery.

(5) Which of the following is a risk factor for tongue cancer?
(a) human papilloma virus types 16 and 18
(b) smoking and chewing tobacco
(c) oral candidiasis
(d) alcohol consumption
(e) consumption of fluoridated water

(6) *True or False*: Dysphagia is rarely observed in clients who have a glossectomy.

(7) *True or False*: Many of the speech compensations used by clients with glossectomy are naturally acquired.

(8) *True or False*: Where a carcinoma of the tongue is at an advanced stage, additional surgical procedures (e.g. mandibulectomy) may need to be performed.

(9) Which of the following techniques is used to assess speech and swallowing in the client with a glossectomy?
(a) electropalatography
(b) nasometry
(c) electroglottography
(d) electromyography
(e) videofluoroscopy

(10) Which of the following statements characterizes the origin of the speech disorder in a client with a glossectomy?
(a) The speech disorder has a neurogenic origin.
(b) The speech disorder has a structural origin.
(c) The speech disorder has a functional origin.
(d) The speech disorder has a neurogenic and functional origin.
(e) The speech disorder has a structural and functional origin.

5.2   Acquired dysarthria

(1) Fill in the blank spaces in these paragraphs using the words in the box below:

A large range of neurological diseases and injuries can cause dysarthria in adults with previously normal speech. The adult who sustains a _____ in a road traffic accident or a violent assault, or who has a stroke may encounter problems with speech production. A formerly healthy adult may develop _____ disorders such as Parkinson's disease, multiple sclerosis or motor _____. In these disorders, difficulties with speech production tend to _____ over time. Different aetiologies demand different forms of assessment and _____ by the speech and language therapist. The client with a rapidly _____ form of motor neurone disease will not regain normal speech function. Before speech declines to the point of unintelligibility, the use of an _____ communication system must be considered. The choice of this system must take full account of the patient's deteriorating physical abilities (e.g. reduced mobility of arms), as well as any _____ and sensory impairments.

In the patient with a stable neurological condition, a realistic treatment goal is the restoration of some degree of premorbid speech production. Assessment may reveal that intelligibility is compromised by deficits in one or more speech _____ subsystems. For example, nasalized consonants and vowels may be related to dysfunction of the _____ port. Weak oral consonants may also be related to velopharyngeal incompetence or may be the result of inadequate _____ support for speech. Intervention may target the range, speed and accuracy of _____ movements for the production of specific speech sounds, for example, the lip closure that is needed to produce bilabial _____ . Where speech impairment is severe and unlikely to respond to treatment by exercises, prosthetic intervention may be required. For example, severe velopharyngeal incompetence may necessitate the use of a _____ lift.

velopharyngeal	stabilize	progressive	palatal
nasals	respiratory	cognitive	head injury
plosives	worsen	neuromuscular	alternative
treatment	psychological	production	prosthetic
neurodegenerative	articulatory	resonatory	neurone disease

(2) Which of the following is *not* associated with acquired dysarthria?
   (a) hypernasal speech related to velopharyngeal incompetence
   (b) limited range and strength of tongue movements
   (c) articulatory groping during attempts to produce a target sound
   (d) greater articulatory difficulty during automatic speech than volitional speech
   (e) phonatory anomalies such as a breathy voice

(3) Which of the following statements characterize dysarthria in the client with Parkinson's disease?
   (a) The client with Parkinson's disease exhibits severe spastic dysarthria.
   (b) The most evident speech feature is excessive speaking volume.
   (c) Laryngeal dysfunction is a prominent feature of dysarthria in Parkinson's disease.
   (d) Dysarthria is rapidly progressive in Parkinson's disease with unintelligibility occurring soon after diagnosis.
   (e) Dysarthria in Parkinson's disease is predominantly hyperkinetic.

(4) *True or False:* Traumatic brain injury is the most common cause of acquired dysarthria in adults.

(5) *True or False:* A mixed dysarthria, which is largely ataxic-spastic in nature, occurs in multiple sclerosis.

(6) Which of the following is a feature of flaccid dysarthria?
   (a) increased muscle tone (hypertonia)
   (b) fasciculations
   (c) atrophy
   (d) slowness of movement
   (e) dysphagia

(7) Which of the following speech production difficulties in acquired dysarthria is related to prosody?

(a) A breathy voice which is caused by failure of the vocal folds to adduct normally.

(b) Weak oral consonants which are related to respiratory difficulties.

(c) Primary stress is placed on incorrect words in utterances.

(d) Speech is hypernasal on account of velopharyngeal incompetence.

(e) Articulation problems which are related to limited range and strength of tongue movements.

(8) Complete the blank spaces in the following statements:

(a) In Parkinson's disease, cells which are responsible for the production of the neurotransmitter dopamine in the _____ of the brain are depleted in substantial numbers.

(b) Ataxic dysarthria occurs when there is damage to the _____ and/or the nerve fibres leading to and from it.

(c) In multiple sclerosis, a pathological process known as _____ can interrupt nerve impulse transmission.

(d) Acquired dysarthria can be caused by stroke-induced damage of the primary _____ in the brain.

(e) Iatrogenic dysarthria occurs when _____ inadvertently damages part of the network of nerves that innervate the speech musculature.

(9) Which of the following statements characterize dysarthria in the client with motor neurone disease?

(a) The client with motor neurone disease exhibits hypokinetic dysarthria.

(b) The type of dysarthria changes as motor neurone disease progresses.

(c) A mixed flaccid-spastic dysarthria in motor neurone disease reflects the involvement of upper and lower motor neurones.

(d) Articulation exhibits normal range of movement, but markedly abnormal speed and accuracy of movement.

(e) The dysarthria stabilizes within six months of the diagnosis of motor neurone disease.

(10) Which of the following statements characterize SLT intervention in clients with rapidly progressive neurodegenerative disorders?

(a) Intervention must address the use of an alternative communication system.

(b) Intervention should aim to improve the intelligibility of the client's speech.

(c) Intervention must aim to establish a safe (non-oral) method of feeding for the client.

(d) Intervention should not consider the communication needs of the ventilator-dependent client.

(e) Physiological exercises that are designed to increase the range and accuracy of the articulators are generally contraindicated in the client with advanced disease.

5.3 Apraxia of speech

(1) Which of the following are *true* statements about apraxia of speech?

(a) Apraxia of speech is a language formulation disorder.

(b) Apraxia of speech can occur alongside oral apraxia.

(c) Apraxia of speech is a motor execution disorder.

(d) Apraxia of speech can occur alongside dysarthria.

(e) Apraxia of speech is a receptive language disorder.

(2) Fill in the blank spaces in this paragraph using the words in the box below:

Apraxia of speech (AOS) is a motor _____ disorder which has an adverse effect on a speaker's intelligibility. Unlike _____ , the disorder does not result from any weakness or paralysis of the speech musculature. However, like dysarthria, the disorder often results from _____ damage caused by a cerebrovascular accident ('stroke') or traumatic event. Volitional speech production is often more difficult for the speaker with AOS than _____ speech production. Also, speech errors are more common as the _____ of words and utterances increases. Often, the speaker with AOS can engage in articulatory _____ as he or she struggles to position the articulators for speech production. The sequencing of muscle movements for speech production is compromised as is the production of consonants and _____ . AOS is often found alongside _____ and dysarthria in adults making a _____ diagnosis of the disorder difficult.

automatic	aphasia	execution	
radiological	vowels	dysarthria	
limb apraxia	differential	groping	
programming	grammatical complexity	phonation	
length	stuttering	voice	neurological

(3) Which of the following are *false* statements about apraxia of speech?
   (a) Mistiming of laryngeal movements can result in voicing errors.
   (b) Speech errors are consistent across multiple productions of the same target.
   (c) Anticipatory phonemic errors occur in apraxia of speech.
   (d) Atrophy is a consistent feature of apraxia of speech.
   (e) The transposition of phonemes is a feature of apraxia of speech.

(4) Prosodic disturbances are commonly found in apraxia of speech. Which of the following statements captures these disturbances?
   (a) Speakers with AOS produce syllabic stress errors.
   (b) Speakers with AOS display speech rate anomalies.
   (c) Speakers with AOS increase their rate of speech as they talk.
   (d) Speakers with AOS consistently place primary stress on the initial syllables of words.
   (e) Speakers with AOS display reduced volume during speech production.

(5) *True* or *False*: Vowel duration is longer in speakers with AOS than in normal speakers.

(6) *True* or *False*: Non-speech oral movements should not be assessed in the AOS speaker.

(7) *True* or *False*: The production of monosyllabic and multisyllabic words should be included in an assessment of AOS.

(8) Which of the following factors distinguishes AOS from dysarthria in adults?
   (a) Only in AOS are speech errors influenced by the linguistic features of utterances.
   (b) Sound substitutions and distortions only occur in AOS.
   (c) Only in dysarthria is there weakness or paralysis of the musculature.
   (d) An automatic-volitional distinction in speech production only occurs in dysarthria.

(e) Only in AOS are speech movements limited on account of neuromuscular weakness.

(9) Fill in the blank spaces in this paragraph using the words in the box below:

An assessment of AOS should include perceptual, acoustic and instrumental techniques. The _____ of speech to the listener is the cornerstone of assessment. The clinician will want to assess the speaker's production, repetition and sequencing of speech sounds in a range of contexts including in words of _____ length and in _____ trials with the same word. Acoustic and _____ assessment of speech can be used to examine the pathophysiological basis of perceived speech anomalies. For example, the perception of slow speech _____ may be shown to be related to the increased _____ of vowel sounds during an acoustic assessment of speech. Similarly, the substitution and distortion of _____ sounds may be related to the mistiming of phonatory activity in the _____ or to the incoordination of _____ valving with tongue movements, both of which can be determined by means of an instrumental assessment of speech. The combination of perceptual, _____ and instrumental approaches to assessment not only results in an accurate _____ of AOS, but is also a rational basis for intervention. In this way, if acoustic assessment reveals a delay in the _____ of voicing as the cause of voicing errors in a speaker with AOS, this delay can then become a target of intervention.

palatal	multiple	onset	nasal cavity
consonant	increasing	phrasing	diagnosis
instrumental	larynx	acoustic	duration
velopharyngeal	decreasing	perception	prolongation
vowel	rate	assessment	respiration

(10) Which of the following statements apply to the treatment of speakers with AOS?
   (a) Treatment should increase the strength and range of articulatory movements.
   (b) Treatment should always prioritize speech-based goals.
   (c) Treatment should consider augmentative and alternative forms of communication.
   (d) Treatment should employ biofeedback from instrumental techniques.
   (e) Treatment should terminate when there is 50% intelligibility of speech to familiar listeners.

Section B: Data analysis exercises

5.4   Glossectomy

Background

Barry and Timmermann (1985) studied seven patients who underwent partial glossectomy for the treatment of carcinoma of the tongue. Surgery in these patients, who were aged 32 to 62 years, ranged from removal of two-thirds of the tongue to removal of a small part of tongue tissue. In some patients, additional surgical procedures were performed including partial removal of the jaw or fixation of the tongue body to the floor of the mouth. These patients, who were all German speakers, received an assessment of their speech. A narrow phonetic transcription of some of their single-word productions is given below.

Target word	Meaning	Phonemic norm	Client production
stritten	quarrelled	/ˈʃtʁɪtən/	[ˈʁˑɪʔn]
Nordwind	north wind	/ˈnɔːtvɪnt/	[ˈnɔːʔvɪnʔ]
stärkere	stronger	/ˈʃtɛəkəʁə/	[ˈfpɛˑχˑʁə]
warmen	warm	/ˈvaːmən/	[ˈvaˑmə̃m]
Mantel	overcoat	/ˈmantəl/	[ˈmantəl]
gehüllt	wrapped	/gəˈhYlt/	[ɣəˈɦYlʔ]
einig	united	/ˈaenɪç/	[ˈaɪnɪə]
stärkeren	stronger	/ˈʃtɛəkəʁən/	[ˈʃpɛʁəʁn]
Weges	way	/ˈveːgəs/	[ˈveˑɣəs]
daherkam	came along	/daˈheəkaːm/	[ʃaˈɦɛəxam]

Exercise 1 The plosive sounds /t, d/ are not used by these speakers. What sounds take their place? Why are these glossectomy speakers performing these substitutions?

Exercise 2 The plosive sounds /k, g/ are not used by these speakers either. However, this time they are not substituted by other plosives. What sounds take the place of velar plosives, and what do these sounds suggest about the articulations these speakers are attempting?

Exercise 3 Three articulatory features are evident in the production of the initial consonant in 'daherkam'. What are these three features?

Exercise 4 How do these speakers produce consonant clusters that contain /t/? The alveolar place of articulation is also problematic for nasal sounds. Give <u>one</u> example of this in the data.

Exercise 5 These speakers make other attempts to replace problematic lingual articulations with other articulations. Describe these attempts in the productions below. The second production is from a speaker whose tongue tip remained mobile but who had relative immobility of the tongue body. Use this information to explain the speaker's articulation.

(a) 'stärkere' [ˈfpɛˑχˑʁə]
(b) 'einig' [ˈaɪnɪə]

5.5   Acquired dysarthria 1

Background

Dysarthria is a motor speech disorder that can occur in children and adults. Its effect on the intelligibility of speech can be highly varied. The assessment of dysarthric speech is increasingly making use of a range of acoustic and physiological techniques (e.g. video-fluoroscopy). However, perceptual assessment that proceeds on the basis of phonetic transcription is still the mainstay of assessment. Typically, transcription proceeds on the basis of single-word productions elicited through testing. Less commonly, spontaneous speech may also be phonetically transcribed.

Task 1

Subject C is a 41-year-old female with multiple sclerosis (MS) who was studied by Ball et al. (2009). C was 21 years of age when she received her MS diagnosis. At that time, she went into a coma for a period of six months. Post-coma, her condition deteriorated rapidly. She now exhibits reduced speech intelligibility, locomotor and general muscular deficits and myodesopsia (floaters). C displays spasticity of the muscles and unilateral paralysis of oral structures, which causes sagging and drooling. Her MS is now of the secondary progressive type. Several of C's utterances in spontaneous conversation underwent narrow phonetic transcription. Two are presented below:

(a) C: I'll ask you a few questions [kw̃ẽʔn̩s] (0.25 s) questions [kwɛst͡ʃn̩s]
(b) C: it runs too fast? [ɨʔ.ɹʌ̃n̩ʂu.fæs]

Task 2

A word intelligibility test was used by Kent et al. (1989) to examine a number of acoustic–phonetic contrasts in the speech of 13 men with amyotrophic lateral sclerosis (ALS). These men displayed dysarthria of varying degrees of severity ranging from almost no impairment to severe impairment (intelligibility scores for these 13 patients ranged from 44% to 99%). The phonetic contrasts which displayed the greatest disruption are shown below for two groups of ALS speakers:

ALS speakers 60–95% intelligible:	high–low
	voiced–voiceless consonants (syllable initial)
	alveolar–palatal fricatives
	stop–nasal
	initial glottal–null
	initial cluster–singleton
ALS speakers < 60% intelligible:	high–low
	voiced–voiceless consonants (syllable initial)
	alveolar–palatal fricatives
	stop–fricative
	stop–nasal
	initial glottal–null
	initial cluster–singleton
	/r/–/w/

A multiple-word intelligibility test and a paired-word intelligibility test were used to examine these phonetic contrasts. In the former test, the first word in a list of four differed from each of the remaining words along a specific phonetic contrast. In the latter test, three word pairs were used which all differed according to one phonetic contrast. The paired-word intelligibility test was used with ALS speakers with severe dysarthria. Stimulus items from both tests are shown below:

Multiple-word intelligibility test:	(a) bad–bed–bat–pad
	(b) sip–ship–tip–zip
	(c) spit–pit–sit–it
	(d) knot–dot–nod–nut
	(e) sigh–shy–tie–thigh
	(f) pit–pet–pat–bit
Paired-word intelligibility test:	(a) bee–pea do–two goo–coo
	(b) add–at buzz–bus need–neat
	(c) eat–it gas–guess pop–pup
	(d) see–tea sew–toe do–zoo
	(e) high–eye hit–it has–as
	(f) way–ray row–woe won–run

Exercise 1 Subject C undertakes a self-repair of the word 'questions' in (a) in Task 1. Which two phonetic features present in the first production of 'questions' are absent in the repaired form of this word?

Exercise 2 In utterance (b) in Task 1, subject C's speech displays a number of phonetic anomalies including zero closure at the end of words and minimal contact for plosive sounds. Using the narrow phonetic transcription provided, give an example of both these anomalies.

Exercise 3 The two groups of ALS speakers both have problems with the following phonetic contrasts. Give one example of a stimulus item from the intelligibility tests which would examine each phonetic contrast.

(a) high–low
(b) voiced–voiceless consonants (syllable initial)
(c) alveolar–palatal fricatives
(d) stop–nasal
(e) initial glottal–null
(f) initial cluster–singleton

Exercise 4 Only ALS speakers who are less than 60% intelligible have significant difficulty with the following phonetic contrasts: stop–fricative and /r/–/w/. Which of the stimulus items in the intelligibility tests assess these contrasts?

Exercise 5 Which phonetic contrast is examined by the word pair 'spit–it'?

5.5   Acquired dysarthria 2

The speech features of acquired dysarthria can vary widely across the dimensions of articulation, resonation, respiration, phonation and prosody. The following case studies describe the speech production abilities of three adults with acquired dysarthria who were studied by Grunwell and Huskins (1979). The dysarthrias of these clients, which are of mixed, ataxic and hypokinetic types, are related to different neuropathologies. Examine the details of each case and then answer the questions below.

Case A: Man aged 39 years with mixed dysarthria

This client, who had a history of hypertension, suffered a cerebrovascular accident (intracerebral haematoma). This resulted in a right-sided weakness with right upper and lower facial weakness, some dysphasia, dysphonia and dysarthria, the latter of brainstem origin. This client's wife had reported that he had somewhat nasal speech even before his CVA and that this had sometimes made him difficult to understand. Over a year after his CVA, his speech musculature was bilaterally affected, but particularly so on the right. There was spastic weakness of his lips and tongue. The client's palate appeared atrophied and foreshortened and this was attributed to flaccid weakness. All articulator movements, but especially those of the palate, were impaired. Given the presence of both bulbar and suprabulbar signs, the client's diagnosis was one of mixed dysarthria.

The client's speech was characterized by a general slow rate which was on account of the very slow movement of all articulators. A continually present phonatory deviation was breathy voice. There was a lack of variation in both the loudness (monoloudness) and pitch of the voice, as well as abnormally high pitch (high monopitch). Speech displayed excessive nasal resonance (hypernasality) and there was audible nasal emission. Articulatory imprecision was a significant characteristic of speech, producing errors in vowel quality and, in terms of consonants, fricative stricture instead of a stop. The client made uneconomical use of the pulmonary airstream leading him to speak in short phrases. The normal patterns of stress, rhythm and intonation were disrupted. The client's increased muscular effort when speaking exacerbated his spasticity, which further contributed to the unintelligibility of his speech.

Case B: Woman aged 27 years with ataxic dysarthria

This client experienced a large post-fossa cerebellar haematoma which was caused by a bleed from an angioma (a vascular malformation which can suddenly rupture). The haematoma was successfully evacuated and the client made a good recovery. She used a wheelchair when she was first admitted to speech therapy due to severe ataxia. She also had ataxic dysarthria. The right side of her body was more impaired than the left side.

The client's speech was slow and exhibited excessive rhythmicity. At both word and phrase levels, stress patterns were aberrant and involved the 'strengthening' of unstressed vowels and a lack of adequate stress prominence. Monopitch and monoloudness resulted from very restricted ranges in the prosodic systems of intonation and loudness. At the level of articulation, most speech was accurate with instances of extremely slow and imprecise movements which affected vowels and consonants. Although the dominant deviation was the abnormal rhythm of speech (scanning speech), there was also muscular weakness with all affected muscle groups fatiguing rapidly. This weakness resulted in the reduced range and force of movement. Phonatory, resonatory and articulatory incoordination resulted in frequent errors in the phonetic features of voicing, aspiration and nasality.

Case C: Man aged 53 years with hypokinetic dysarthria

This client had a history of Parkinson's disease which first manifested as clumsiness of the left hand. A pallidectomy was performed which had succeeded in reducing his tremor and improving his speech. However, subsequently, he needed amplification of his voice. After speech therapy, his voice improved but he was nonetheless forced to resign from his job. A neurologist prescribed L-dopa, and he remained physically active. Later, he was referred again to speech therapy. At this time, his speech was extremely rapid and unintelligible, although his voice was still audible.

The most significant feature of this client's speech was his extremely rapid rate of utterance. This was related to the abnormally accelerated movement of the articulators. There was often imprecision of articulatory gestures. An irregularity in the timing of segments was revealed on spectrographic analysis, with glides and consonants lengthened and vowels shortened. There was a lack of variation in stress, intonation and loudness. An uncontrolled repetition of articulatory movements was observed on occasion. Erratic syllable structure and incorrect word rhythm were related to irregularity in the temporal distribution of segments.

Exercise 1 Which of the following are *true* statements about the mixed dysarthria of the male client in Case A?

(a) This client displays inefficient glottal and velopharyngeal valving of the pulmonary airstream, leading to increased effort in speech production as a means of compensation.

(b) The client's hypernasal speech post-CVA reflects in part premorbid features of speech production.

(c) The client is able to reach articulatory target positions but does so slowly.

(d) The client's breathy voice is related to a failure of the vocal folds to abduct normally.

(e) The client's prosodic disturbances are related to the lack of variation in pitch and loudness as well as to a lack of control over breath flow.

Exercise 2 Name one bulbar sign and one suprabulbar sign which contributed to the diagnosis of mixed dysarthria in Case A.

Exercise 3 Two neuromuscular deficits – ataxia and hypotonia – are evident in the dysarthria of the client in Case B. Describe one way in which each of these deficits is manifested in the speech of this client.

Exercise 4 Which of the following statements characterize the aberrant rhythmic structure of the speech of the client in Case B?

(a) Excessive rhythmicity is a form of over compensation for the client's lack of coordination of neuromuscular speech events.

(b) On spectrographic analysis, this client's rhythmicity will appear as 'segment timing' or the equal lengths of vowels and consonants.

(c) Excessive rhythmicity in this client's speech is an attempt on her part to compensate for muscular weakness.

(d) Excessive rhythmicity can be expected to have a minimal effect on the intelligibility of the client's speech.

(e) Unstressed syllables can be expected to be unaffected by the excessive rhythmicity of this client's speech.

Exercise 5 Respond with *true* or *false* to each of the following statements about the speech of the client in Case C:

(a) This client's rapid rate of utterance is symptomatic of a Parkinsonian clinical feature called festination.

(b) Unintelligibility is related to a lack of coordination of movements for speech.

(c) Reduced vocal intensity is typical of the dysarthria seen in Parkinson's disease.

(d) Articulatory movements are very slow and have a reduced range.

(e) This client's uncontrolled repetition of articulatory movements is known as palilalia.

5.5   Acquired dysarthria 3

Wilson's disease is a rare, inherited, metabolic disorder in which the body is unable to process dietary copper. The resultant deposits of copper in the brain (copper is also deposited in the liver and cornea) can cause neurological damage, which is permanent if treatment of the disease is delayed. A mixed ataxic-hypokinetic-spastic dysarthria is a feature of the disease. Day and Parnell (1987) treated an adult male ('R') with the disease over a ten-year period. Examine the details of this case and then answer the questions below.

Case study: 35-year-old male with Wilson's disease

History and presenting symptoms: R first began to experience dysarthria, dysphagia, drooling, decreased mental function and some dystonia at 23 years of age. Other neurological signs and behavioural changes, which were exhibited later, included right foot drop, clumsiness in the upper extremities, postural changes and marked personality changes (e.g. intermittent periods of depression). R had an older sister who had been diagnosed two years earlier with Wilson's disease. She died shortly thereafter. Following diagnosis of Wilson's disease, R failed to comply with the medical regimen prescribed by his doctor. He underwent a 18-month period of psychiatric treatment for depression. During the same year, he was hospitalized in a mental health facility after attempting suicide by drug overdose. His first marriage failed during this time.

Pre-treatment speech: The psychiatrist who had treated R for his depression noted that his 'speech (had) deteriorated almost to the point of being completely non-understandable' and that 'the chances of significant improvement (were) poor'. At his first attendance at a speech pathology clinic, R was observed to be profoundly dysarthric and his speech was non-functional. He relied heavily on sign language and written messages in his communication, neither of which was particularly effective on account of R's poor manual motor control. Drooling, dysphagia, oral and facial rigidity and weakness and a fixed, grimace-like expression were also noted at this session.

Speech intervention: Early efforts to achieve greater precision and flexibility of oral structure movement through oral-motor exercises produced no significant gain and were rapidly abandoned. Similarly, there was no noticeable improvement in intelligibility as a result of attempts to increase vocal volume and differentiate vowel productions. The production of single consonants and consonant clusters became a focus of intervention for a period of several years. Significantly reduced ratings of R's intelligibility were associated with his particularly difficult production of multisyllabic words and final-position consonants. Self-monitoring of R's productions was encouraged, while his reliance on ineffective gestural communication was discouraged. The use of augmentative and alternative communication was consistently rejected by R during therapy.

General 'suprasegmental' guidelines were implemented in therapy over the accurate production of individual sounds (the latter was judged to produce minimal gains for the intelligibility of connected speech). These guidelines were: (1) slowed rate, (2) syllable-by-syllable production, (3) overarticulation and (4) increased mouth opening. The combined effect of these guidelines on the intelligibility of R's speech was so significant that R was able to secure part-time employment for the first time since his diagnosis. Supplemental work on adequate respiratory support, appropriate pausing, and effective use of stress and intonation patterns failed to have as great an impact on the intelligibility of R's speech as that which was achieved by slowed rate and syllable-by-syllable production. It was observed that R's motor speech abilities were particularly vulnerable to the effects of fatigue. Given the detrimental effects of fatigue on R's speech production, he was encouraged to adjust his daily activities to ensure he received sufficient sleep, particularly in advance of therapy sessions. Because R did not respond cooperatively to this recommendation, his compliance with this request was made a precondition on his subsequent re-enrolment for treatment.

Traditional therapy techniques were ineffective in improving R's velopharyngeal closure and reducing the hypernasality of his speech. However, after wearing a palatal lift appliance for nearly two years, the hypernasality of R's speech had markedly decreased, even in the absence of wearing the appliance. These gains in velopharyngeal function were maintained over time, with R only resorting to using the palatal lift when fatigue interfered with his speech.

Although R was able to achieve increased speech intelligibility in the clinic, he persistently failed to generalize these gains to communication in a range of other settings. He was given increased responsibility for the self-evaluation of his intelligibility and compensatory guidelines both in and out of the clinic, with the latter involving the completion of daily logs by R and his communicative partners. R subsequently remarried. His second wife attended occasional therapy sessions in order to discuss objectives and recommendations and learn how to implement techniques at home. With the greater participation of R's wife in terms of providing support, feedback and behaviour management, it was hoped that R could be discharged from therapy.

Exercise 1 A mixed ataxic-hypokinetic-spastic dysarthria is a clinical feature of Wilson's disease. This dysarthria results from lesions to several brain structures. Select the structures in question from the list below.

(a) upper motor neurones
(b) hypothalamus
(c) basal ganglia
(d) cerebellum
(e) lower motor neurones

Exercise 2 R's dysarthria is particularly severe and involves impairment in each of the speech production subsystems. Give <u>one</u> example of how R's speech is compromised in each of the following subsystems.

(a) articulation
(b) respiration
(c) resonation
(d) phonation
(e) prosody

Exercise 3 During intervention, R was encouraged to comply with a number of 'supraseg-mental' guidelines which had a particularly positive effect on the intelligibility of his speech. Two in particular, slowed rate and syllable-by-syllable production, appeared to be especially effective. Explain how both these techniques achieved an increase in the intelligibility of R's speech.

Exercise 4 Management of R's velopharyngeal dysfunction involved the use of a palatal lift appliance. Which of the following statements characterize R's velopharyngeal dysfunction and its management?

(a) R's velopharyngeal dysfunction has a structural origin.
(b) The improvement in R's velopharyngeal function over time can be explained by the non-stable nature of his neurological disorder.
(c) R's velopharyngeal dysfunction is likely to be related to the presence of an excessively capacious pharynx.
(d) A palatal lift succeeded in R's case because his soft palate retained some mobility, but not enough to make the full excursion required to make contact with the pharyngeal wall.
(e) R's velopharyngeal dysfunction has a neurogenic origin.

Exercise 5 R's medical management and speech intervention are compromised on more than one occasion. What factor is responsible for this compromise? Is this factor likely to be a premorbid characteristic of R or a clinical feature of his neurological disorder?

5.6   Apraxia of speech

Data 1

La Pointe and Johns (1975) examined articulatory performance in 13 adults who developed apraxia of speech after sustaining cortical damage through a CVA or trauma. The mean time since onset was 12.15 months (range = 1–35 months). The sequential nature of these subjects' articulatory errors was examined in detail. Three types of sequential error were identified: anticipatory, reiterative and metathesis. An error was classified as anticipatory if a phoneme was replaced by one that occurred later in the word. If a phoneme was replaced by one that occurred earlier in the word, the error was classified as reiterative. If two phonemes switched places within a word, the error was classified as metathesis. Several sequential errors produced by the subjects in this study are shown in the table below.

	Target word	Client production
(a)	sandwich	'wansin – sanwich'
(b)	yellow	'redul, ledul, (pause) lelo'
(c)	dress	'dred'
(d)	grasshopper	'grap – popper, let's see, – grass – hopper'
(e)	December	'ees, ees, esender'
(f)	telephone	'teflone – tefalone'
(g)	bicycle	'b – bai – bai – s – s – sai – s – uh – bai – sikl'

Data 2

The following 15 features of acquired apraxia of speech are taken from the *Apraxia Battery for Adults* (Dabul, 2000):

(1) Exhibits phonemic anticipatory errors.
(2) Exhibits phonemic perseverative errors.
(3) Exhibits phonemic transposition errors.
(4) Exhibits phonemic voicing errors.
(5) Exhibits phonemic vowel errors.
(6) Exhibits visible/audible searching.
(7) Exhibits numerous off-target attempts at the word.
(8) Errors are highly inconsistent.
(9) Errors increase as phonemic sequence increases.
(10) Exhibits fewer errors with automatic speech than volitional speech.
(11) Exhibits marked difficulty initiating speech.
(12) Intrudes schwa sound /ə/ between syllables or in consonant clusters.
(13) Exhibits abnormal prosodic features.
(14) Exhibits awareness of errors and inability to correct them.
(15) Exhibits expressive-receptive gap.

Dronkers (1996) presents the following speech output of two speakers with apraxia of speech:

Patient H.F. (attempting to say 'cushion'): 'Oh, uh, uh, chookun uh, uh, uh, dook, I know what it's called, it's c-u, uh, no, it's, it's chook chookun, no'.

Patient D.B. (repeating 'catastrophe' five times): 'catastrophe, patastrofee, t, catastrophe, katasrifrobee, aw sh-, ka, kata, sh-, sh-. I do not know'.

Exercise 1 For each production in Data 1, indicate if the speaker has committed an anticipatory, reiterative or metathesis error.

Exercise 2 Which of Dabul's apraxia of speech (AOS) characteristics in Data 2 is exemplified by the following speech errors?

(a) pep for 'pet'
(b) moan for 'man'
(c) lelo for 'yellow'
(d) Arifca for 'Africa'
(e) ben for 'pen'

Exercise 3 In attempting to say 'cushion', patient H.F. in Data 2 says 'chookun . . . dook . . . chookun'. Which of Dabul's AOS characteristics are exemplified by this speech behaviour?

Exercise 4 Which of Dabul's AOS characteristics captures the following speech behaviour exhibited by patient H.F.? 'I know what it's called, it's c-u . . . no . . . chookun, no'.

Exercise 5 In his production of 'catastrophe', patient D.B. produces 'patastrofee' and 'katas-rifrobee'. In terms of syllable structure, how would you characterize these errors?

SUGGESTIONS FOR FURTHER READING

Bressmann, T. 2014. 'Head and neck cancer and communication', in L. Cummings (ed.), *Cambridge handbook of communication disorders*, Cambridge: Cambridge University Press, 161–84 (section 10.2 on glossectomy).

Cummings, L. 2008. *Clinical linguistics*, Edinburgh: Edinburgh University Press (sections 5.2 and 5.3).

2014a. *Communication disorders*, Houndmills: Palgrave Macmillan (chapter 4).

Duffy, J. R. 2013. *Motor speech disorders: substrates, differential diagnosis, and management*, third edition, St. Louis, MO: Elsevier Mosby (parts 1 and 2).

Jacks, A. and Robin, D. A. 2013. 'Apraxia of speech', in J. S. Damico, N. Müller and M. J. Ball (eds.), *The handbook of language and speech disorders*, Oxford: Wiley-Blackwell, 391–409.

McNeil, M. R., Robin, D. A. and Schmidt, R. A. 2009. 'Apraxia of speech', in M. R. McNeil (ed.), *Clinical management of sensorimotor speech disorders*, second edition, New York: Thieme, 249–68.

Murdoch, B. E. 2010. *Acquired speech and language disorders: a neuroanatomical and functional neurological approach*, second edition, Chichester: Wiley-Blackwell (chapters 9, 10 and 11).

2014. 'Acquired dysarthria', in L. Cummings (ed.), *Cambridge handbook of communication disorders*, Cambridge: Cambridge University Press, 185–210.

Ogar, J., Slama, H., Dronkers, N., Amici, S. and Gorno-Tempini, M. L. 2005. 'Apraxia of speech: an overview', *Neurocase* **11**:6, 427–32.

Robin, D. A. and Flagmeier, S. 2014. 'Apraxia of speech', in L. Cummings (ed.), *Cambridge handbook of communication disorders*, Cambridge: Cambridge University Press, 211–23.

Chapter 6

Acquired language disorders

Adults can sustain injuries and illnesses which cause disruption of previously intact language skills. Aphasia is the most prominent language disorder which is acquired in adulthood. Typically, it is caused by damage to the language centres in the left hemisphere of the brain following a cerebrovascular accident or stroke. Less common causes of aphasia are traumatic brain injury, brain tumours and cerebral infections. In rare cases, aphasia may result from damage to the right hemisphere of the brain. Aphasias are classified as fluent and non-fluent types. In fluent aphasia, there is effortless spoken output which exhibits the normal suprasegmental features of speech. However, this output often contains copious amounts of jargon (hence, the term 'jargon aphasia') in which neologisms are present. The client with fluent aphasia also has a severe auditory comprehension deficit and displays limited awareness of their communication problems. In non-fluent aphasia, there is reduced, effortful spoken output. The client is aware of, and is often distressed by, their problems with spoken language. Grammatical structure is markedly reduced with content words (e.g. nouns) retained, while function words (e.g. articles) are omitted. This gives speech the appearance of a telegram (hence, the use of the term 'agrammatic aphasia' to describe this type of aphasia).

Damage to the right hemisphere of the brain can cause a different type of language disorder in adults. In so-called right-hemisphere language disorder, structural language skills are largely intact while there are marked impairments of pragmatic and discourse skills. These impairments include the concrete, literal interpretation of figurative language, egocentric discourse which relates the speaker's personal experience, neglect of the hearer's perspective in formulating utterances, and problems with topic management and narrative structure. Many of these communication difficulties appear to be related to cognitive deficits such as executive dysfunction.

Like children, adults may also sustain a traumatic brain injury (TBI). Adults with TBI often pass standardized language batteries and yet exhibit communication impairments which are severe enough to limit occupational functioning and social integration (see Cummings (2011) and chapter 3 in Cummings (2014d) for discussion). These impairments take the form of pragmatic and discourse deficits and are most evident during narrative production and conversation. Finally, language can be impaired in a range of dementias. These include, most notably, Alzheimer's disease. However, the language features of several non-Alzheimer's dementias (e.g. AIDS dementia complex) are increasingly being characterized (see chapter 6 in Cummings (2014d) for discussion).

Section A: Short-answer questions

6.1   Acquired aphasia

(1) Fill in the blank spaces in these paragraphs using the words in the box below:
Aphasia is by far the most extensively examined acquired neurogenic communication disorder in adults. Although several types exist, the two main subtypes of the

disorder are fluent and _____ aphasia. These forms of aphasia are also known by other names such as _____ and Broca's aphasia (referring to the particular anatomical regions of the brain that are compromised) and receptive and _____ aphasia (referring to whether language comprehension and production are compromised, respectively).

The adult with non-fluent aphasia struggles to produce language. Many function words are omitted with the result that speech has the appearance of a telegram. It is for this reason that this form of aphasia is often described as _____ aphasia. While language output is often severely affected, language _____ is relatively intact. The client with non-fluent aphasia is often adept at using stereotypical forms to hold his or her turn in _____ during periods of non-fluency. The speaker with non-fluent aphasia is _____ of his or her expressive difficulties which can lead to considerable frustration. Semantic paraphasic errors are also in evidence, with uttered lexemes bearing a _____ relation to the target word.

The adult with fluent aphasia presents a very different pattern of linguistic deficits. Spoken output is fluent and effortless and the speaker is largely _____ of the severity of his or her communication problems. The comprehension of language is often severely impaired. Meaningless utterances which contain 'new words', or _____, confer a jargon quality on spoken output. It is for this reason that this particular form of aphasia is also known as _____ aphasia. Where short, truncated utterances disrupt prosody in the non-fluent speaker, the effortless production of jargon utterances in fluent aphasia means that the intonational and suprasegmental features of normal speech are largely _____. Lexical retrieval problems are also evident. The client with fluent aphasia may engage in _____, or talk around a word, when he or she is unable to retrieve it. The repeated production of a linguistic form, a behaviour known as _____, is also found in clients with fluent aphasia.

neologisms	phonemic paraphasias	aware	jargon
conduction	comprehension	perseveration	preserved
non-fluent	circumlocution	expressive	telegrammatic
lexical	conversation	Wernicke's	anomic
agrammatic	unaware	anterior aphasia	semantic

(2) *True* or *False*: The term 'aphasia' is applied to all acquired language disorders in adults.

(3) *True* or *False*: Crossed aphasia describes aphasia that is caused by damage to the right hemisphere of the brain.

(4) *True* or *False*: Cerebral infections are not one of the aetiologies of aphasia.

(5) Which of the following statements characterize linguistic deficits in the client with non-fluent aphasia?
   (a) Receptive language problems are more severe than expressive language deficits.
   (b) There are marked prosodic disturbances in language output.
   (c) Linguistic deficits in non-fluent aphasia are related to severe cognitive impairments.
   (d) Linguistic deficits in non-fluent aphasia are largely resistant to therapeutic intervention.

(e) There is a predominance of content words in the output of the speaker with non-fluent aphasia.

(6) Which of the following statements characterize the assessment of clients with aphasia by speech and language therapists?
(a) Cognitive neuropsychological models of language processing have had a significant influence on the assessment of aphasia.
(b) The focus of assessment is on syntactic aspects of language.
(c) Assessment should use a range of formal and informal techniques.
(d) Formal methods of assessment are well suited to an analysis of pragmatic aspects of language.
(e) Conversation analysis has an important role to play in the assessment of conversational skills in the client with aphasia.

(7) Aphasia results from damage to the language centres in the _____ hemisphere of the brain.

(8) Aphasia can affect the reception and expression of spoken, _____ and signed language.

(9) Which of the following statements characterize the treatment of clients with aphasia by speech and language therapists?
(a) The focus of treatment is on the speed, range and accuracy of articulatory gestures for speech.
(b) Treatment should be discontinued at six months post-onset in the case of stroke patients.
(c) Treatment should include the participation of the conversational partners of the person with aphasia.
(d) Treatment should consider the adequacy of respiratory support for speech production.
(e) Treatment should aim to give the severely aphasic client functional communication skills.

(10) Which of the following is a benefit of conducting group therapy with the person with aphasia?
(a) Group therapy provides the person with aphasia with psychological support.
(b) Group therapy closely resembles everyday communication in terms of the number of participants and social dimensions.
(c) Group therapy allows therapists to focus on the social interaction deficits of the person with aphasia.
(d) Group therapy provides opportunities for the generalization of language skills to occur.
(e) Group therapy allows therapists to address the significant cognitive deficits of the person with aphasia.

6.2   Right-hemisphere language disorder

(1) Which of the following is *not* a cause of acquired right-hemisphere damage in adults?
(a) cerebrovascular accident
(b) cerebral palsy

(c) brain tumour

(d) phenylketonuria

(e) traumatic brain injury

(2) Whereas structural language is impaired in the left-hemisphere _____, the language disorder in right-hemisphere damage is characterized by deficits in _____ and discourse.

(3) Which of the following is *not* a feature of right-hemisphere language disorder?

(a) Discourse is tangential and egocentric.

(b) Cerebrovascular accidents are the most common cause of right-hemisphere language disorder.

(c) Comprehension of embedded clauses is impaired.

(d) There is a tendency towards literal interpretation of non-literal language.

(e) There are problems with the appreciation of humour.

(4) Fill in the blank spaces in this paragraph using the words in the box below:

Penelope Myers published the first formal study of discourse-level communication disorders in right-hemisphere damaged adults in 1979. This study arose out of the author's observation that stroke patients with right-hemisphere damage who had intact _____ skills were nevertheless communicating _____. Specifically, these patients produced 'irrelevant and often excessive information' and seemed 'to miss the implication of [a] question and to respond in a most literal and _____ way' (1979: 38). When attempting to respond to open-ended _____, these patients 'wended their way through a maze of disassociated detail, seemingly incapable of filtering out unnecessary _____' (38). The components of a narrative, although available to these patients, could not be correctly assembled. There was difficulty 'in extracting critical bits of information, in seeing the relationships among them, and in reaching conclusions or drawing _____ based on those relationships' (39). Although the detail provided by these patients was related to the general _____, its appearance seemed irrelevant because it had not been 'integrated into a whole' (39). These combined impairments of _____ and discourse compromised the communication of these patients beyond the dysarthria for which they were receiving treatment.

concrete	theme	pragmatics	syntactic
inadequately	topic	semantics	language
inferences	questions	information	implicatures

(5) *True* or *False*: Executive function deficits are present in clients with right-hemisphere damage but are unrelated to pragmatic impairments in this population.

(6) *True* or *False*: There is a relationship between communication impairment in clients with right-hemisphere damage and the ability to generate and manipulate inferences.

(7) *True* or *False*: Theory of mind impairments have been reported in clients with right-hemisphere damage and are related to pragmatic deficits in this population.

(8) Which of the following is a pragmatic deficit in clients with right-hemisphere damage?

(a) impaired confrontation naming
(b) impaired visuospatial skills
(c) impaired comprehension of wh-interrogatives
(d) impaired comprehension of metaphors
(e) impaired set-shifting skills

(9) Researchers have found that adults with right-hemisphere damage have difficulty comprehending sarcasm. This difficulty, they argue, is related to problems in attributing mental states such as communicative _____ to the minds of speakers.

(10) *True or False*: The processing of emotional prosody is intact in adults with right-hemisphere damage.

6.3 Traumatic brain injury

(1) *True or False*: Traumatic brain injury can result in multi-focal cerebral pathology.

(2) *True or False*: The expression 'cognitive communication disorder' reflects the significant role of cognitive deficits in the language impairments of adults who sustain a traumatic brain injury.

(3) Which of the following is *not* a pragmatic-discourse deficit in traumatic brain injury?
(a) difficulty producing indirect requests
(b) difficulty comprehending relative clauses
(c) difficulty understanding sarcasm
(d) difficulty giving procedural steps to a listener on how to play a board game
(e) difficulty in narrative production

(4) The communication disorder in traumatic brain injury has a substantial basis in cognitive deficits which are related to _____ lobe pathology.

(5) Pragmatic and discourse impairments in traumatic brain injury are increasingly being linked to cognitive deficits. These deficits consist largely in impairments of _____ functions and theory of _____ skills.

(6) *True or False*: Repetitiveness is not a feature of narratives produced by clients who sustain a traumatic brain injury.

(7) *True or False*: Topic management skills are normally intact in clients with traumatic brain injury.

(8) Which of the following statements is *true* of language and communication following traumatic brain injury?
(a) Aphasia may be present in the client with traumatic brain injury.
(b) Dysarthria and apraxia of speech are only found in clients with severe traumatic brain injury.
(c) Clients with traumatic brain injury can pass conventional language tests and yet still exhibit significant communication impairments.
(d) Clients with traumatic brain injury are adept at using indirect means (e.g. hints) to make requests.
(e) The content of narratives produced by clients with traumatic brain injury often does not address the informational needs of listeners.

(9) Researchers have found theory of mind impairments in adults with traumatic brain injury. These impairments are believed to account for the difficulty these

adults have in recognizing the communicative _____ which motivate speakers' utterances.

(10) Which of the following is *not* among the neurological sequelae of traumatic brain injury in adults?
 (a) sensory impairments
 (b) epilepsy
 (c) hemiplegia
 (d) hemianopia
 (e) premorbid personality traits

6.4 Dementias

(1) Which of the following conditions is *not* a cause of dementia?
 (a) HIV infection
 (b) Creutzfeldt-Jakob disease
 (c) hyperthyroidism
 (d) cerebrovascular disease
 (e) excessive alcohol consumption

(2) *True* or *False*: Progressive non-fluent aphasia is a type of frontotemporal dementia.

(3) *True* or *False*: Clients with semantic dementia exhibit surface dyslexia.

(4) *True* or *False*: In HIV dementia, pragmatic language skills are intact while structural language skills are severely impaired.

(5) Which of the following is *not* a linguistic feature of progressive non-fluent aphasia?
 (a) agrammatism
 (b) severe dysarthria
 (c) phonemic paraphasias
 (d) anomia
 (e) effortful speech

(6) Which of the following is a linguistic feature of semantic dementia?
 (a) fluent, empty speech
 (b) severe anomia
 (c) semantic paraphasias
 (d) accelerated speech rate
 (e) glossomania

(7) The progression to mutism in progressive non-fluent aphasia necessitates consideration of _____ and _____ communication devices early in the course of the disease.

(8) Studies have shown that language subsystems are not uniformly impaired in Alzheimer's disease. Deterioration in _____ and pragmatic knowledge occurs relatively early in the course of the disease, while impairments in syntax and _____ occur later in the condition.

(9) *True* or *False*: Lewy body disease dementia is the most common form of dementia in people above 65 years of age.

(10) *True* or *False*: Aphasia, alexia and agraphia are typically absent in HIV dementia.

Section B: Data analysis exercises

6.5   Acquired aphasia 1

Background

The following extracts of data have been produced by adults with fluent aphasia (Chapman et al., 1998). The data was collected during a range of discourse production tasks. The tasks involved (a) retelling fables, (b) capturing the gist of fables, (c) conveying the lesson of fables, (d) story generation based on a single frame picture, and (e) verbal explanations of the meaning of proverbs. Each of these tasks places different demands on a speaker's cognitive, linguistic and pragmatic skills. Examine each extract and then answer the questions below.

Fable retelling

Subjects read and heard the following fable, which they were then required to retell:

A hungry raven saw that pigeons in the pigeon coop had a lot of food. He painted his feathers white to look like them. But when he started to crow, they realized that he was a raven and chased him away. So he returned to his own kind. But the other ravens did not recognize him because he had his feathers painted white, so they also chased him away.

Extract 1

A raven saw a, saw the patg- (6 seconds) (Examiner: pigeons) pigeon, pigeons in the ka-coop. The-the raven looked and they had of food. The raven where he got th-th-th uh paint to paint his feathers white so he can go into the cope-coop and have some food then. Well he got in there, into the coop and as soon as he wanted foo, no he-he wanted to, not talk, well he wanted to crow. The pigeon, 'No-ho, that's not a cousin'. So they threw him out and he had to run away. And then he went back to the raven-raven family and-and they looked at him, his color isn't right. It was white so he had to lea- they threw him out.

Gist of fables

Subjects were required to capture the main idea or gist of a fable.

Extract 2

Don't change, or like that? Don't change the color . . . don't change, don't change your, don't change, don't change yourself, what you are to get some money, *** to get uh food.

Lesson of fables

Subjects were asked to convey a lesson which could be learned from a fable.

Extract 3

Don't change, don't change, don't change, don't change things to, don't-don't-don't take, don't take, don't change, don't change your life just to get what you want to.

Story generation

Subjects were shown a single-frame, contextually rich picture. They were asked to observe the picture, and generate a story based on it. The story was related to the examiner while the picture was face down. The picture was a Norman Rockwell print which depicted a rural scene around the 1930s. The picture displays an older man dressed in work clothes who is smoking a rolled cigarette. There is a young man dressed in a suit. He has a small wrapped parcel, books and a suitcase, the latter with a State U. sticker on it. There is also a sheep dog with his head on the young man's lap. Both men are sitting next to each other on the running board of an old truck.

Extract 4

Let's see, it must have been during the 1930s uh a young man going to college, university, state university. And they were sitting on a a kind of a, on a small, on a ru-ru-rubber, rubber, rudder, sitting on a rubber of a car. They used to have that. And uh this uh, there was a, this young man he has a friend, a friend which was a dog, probably sheep-shep-shepard. And dad was smoking and he was thinking well, 'you've got to say goodbye'. And uh I think he was a farmer. And so the man is thinking, 'I'm going to leave and going to college or in the university'. And dad is gonna wis-miss and so will the dog miss this young man.

Proverb meaning

Subjects were asked to explain the meaning of the proverb 'One swallow doesn't make a summer'.

Extract 5

All right, (laughs) so what does that mean, um, well it takes all summer. Uh, what, uh, well, a swallow doesn't make a summer. Right. Um, it takes time, uh let's see time, uh, autumn could also be just as well, so the swallow, what about it, if he goes in the summer time, well, that's great, but um, how about in the autumn, he goes south. I'm not doing well with this at all. I mean it doesn't um, I don't know, maybe the birds, uh, one swallow, that's a bird isn't it? (Examiner: Can you think of a reason why one swallow wouldn't make a summer?) Right. Nope. I'm sorry.

Exercise 1 A number of linguistic problems compromise the discourse performance of the subjects in the above extracts. These problems include phonemic paraphasias and semantic paraphasias. Provide two examples of each type of linguistic difficulty.

Exercise 2 What linguistic features of the extracts indicate that these subjects have word-finding problems? Provide three examples.

Exercise 3 Some extracts have higher informational content than other extracts. Indicate which extracts have the highest informational content, and suggest why this is the case.

Exercise 4 Some extracts have lower informational content than other extracts. Indicate which extracts have the lowest informational content, and suggest why this is the case.

Exercise 5 Much can be gleaned about the cognitive skills of these subjects with fluent aphasia. Which of the following are *true* statements about those skills?

(a) The subjects display intact theory of mind skills.
(b) The subjects display limited awareness of their linguistic and communicative difficulties.
(c) The subjects display intact memory processes.
(d) The subjects display impaired attention processes.
(e) During story generation, the subject displays poor planning and organization.

6.5   Acquired aphasia 2

Background

Adults with Wernicke's aphasia produce a number of distinctive linguistic errors in their spoken output. Some clients with this language disorder can produce copious amounts of jargon. This can take the form of real words, which are linked together in ways that do not make sense, or it can involve the creation of new words (neologisms). As well as the production of jargon, adults with Wernicke's aphasia can produce errors called semantic paraphasias. In these errors, there is a semantic relationship between the actual word that the client utters and the target word. Both types of error are evident in the data below from two adults with Wernicke's aphasia.

Hough (1993) describes the case of a 66-year-old female who suffered two left-hemisphere strokes. This woman's language difficulties were documented over a ten-month period following the onset of these strokes. She received a diagnosis of Wernicke's aphasia which was characterized by neologistic jargon and a severe auditory comprehension deficit. Eight months post-stroke, no linguistic or communicative improvements had been observed. A new therapeutic regimen was then introduced. After just two months, the naming abilities of the patient improved as did her general ability to communicate in conversation. The table below contains the naming responses of this woman on items in the Boston Naming Test (BNT) and the Boston Diagnostic Aphasia Examination (BDAE) at different intervals post-stroke. These responses are characterized by neologistic and semantic jargon.

Data 1

	At onset	7 mths post-onset	8 mths post-onset	10 mths post-onset
BNT:				
'scissors'	/ækwʌb/	/fwɛno/	/saɪbwɚ/	/kʌtmæn/
'flower'	/lɛdi/	/wide/	/fenhal/	/blumpat/
'pencil'	/kwobɚ/	/bɪvɪk/	/gɪfku/	/pɛnres/
BDAE:				
'drinking'	/pɛpo/	/kɪbin/	/nodɪk/	/kʌpʌp/
'cactus'	/kæbat/	/tukɪt/	/sʌtʌs/	/prɪkəl/

Background

The data below was obtained from a 74-year-old right-handed woman, known as JT, who was studied by Buckingham (HWB) and Rekart (1979). JT sustained a left parietal cerebrovascular accident. Her clinical symptoms were typical of Wernicke's aphasia. JT produced neologistic jargon and exhibited impaired verbal comprehension, reading and writing. Her spoken output was recorded over an eight-month period at regular intervals between two and three weeks. Some of the utterances presented below were produced during spontaneous speech; others were produced during picture identification, repetition and the reading aloud of isolated words. The target word is indicated in brackets.

Data 2

Picture and body part identification

(1) (cactus) 'Well this is [fil] down in the [narəi] (south)...'
(2) (bicycle) 'I used to run (ride) one. Oh, I used to love to ride it!'
(3) (pretzels) 'Well, it's a drink (eat) 'em with coffee...you break 'em up and chew 'em up when you're drinking with coffee...Yeah, but I don't eat 'em too much...'
(4) (triangle) 'That's a [kɔkeik] isn't it? Cake. A [radʒ] or what is that? There's cookie case.'
(5) (knuckles) 'Well, that's the fingers...'
(6) (shoulder) 'My mouth...my neck...'

Conversation

(7)

> HWB: It's hot outside.
> JT: It wasn't cold (hot) for me. I had to close the [wɪnər]...
> the girl (nurse) said I had to put the [hjurər] on...it was cold in here...
> and you said it was hot.

(8)

> JT: This is apples. My brother brought me an apple today...(her brother holds up an apple)
> HWB: Cherry
> JT: Cherry. That's what I meant.

(9)

> HWB: Green
> JT: What?
> HWB: Green
> JT: Well, that doesn't look red to me!
> HWB: No, green
> JT: That's looks to me it's red
> HWB: No, this is green
> JT: That's [gri]...but it must be I didn't say it

(10)

> HWB: What's today?
> JT: Three o'clock

Other utterances

(11) 'I would be able to hear you better with that than this eye (ear)...'

(12) 'Well, my wife (husband) had a couple other brothers'

(13) 'Well the first one lived in – uh – down on the north (south)...'; 'They don't come down (up)... He'll come up after it's colder...' (JT is referring to her son who lives in Florida)

(14) 'I have two daughters (sons) children'

(15) '...she's a policeman woman'

(16) 'I can see (hear) you talking that way...'

(17) 'My brother (sister) he's dead...'

(18) 'Well, this is a little girl boy...'

(19) '...we early January... they wake you up so early!'

(20) 'They're too big! They're too big! They gotta make bigger for my feet... my shoes are little aren't big enough'

Exercise 1   In Data set 1, there is a significant transition in the naming abilities of this Wernicke's aphasic client following the introduction of a new treatment approach at eight months post-stroke. Using this client's single-word productions as evidence, describe the transition that occurs.

Exercise 2   In Data set 2, JT's semantic paraphasic errors involve words from several semantic fields. Identify nine such fields and give an example of a semantic paraphasic error from each one.

Exercise 3   Using examples, list four grammatical categories to which JT's substitutions belong. Are JT's substitutions changing or preserving the grammatical category of the target word?

Exercise 4   The substitutions that JT has made can be characterized in terms of the following lexical relations. Give one example of each lexical relation in JT's data.

(a) gradable antonymy
(b) meronymy
(c) multiple incompatibility
(d) hyponymy

Exercise 5   There are a number of other interesting features in JT's data. To encourage you to think about them, answer the following questions. Provide evidence for your answer in each case.

(a) Does JT produce phonemic paraphasic errors in her spoken output?
(b) Is JT able to cue herself into the use of the target form after she has used a substitution?
(c) Are any of JT's substitutions motivated by a visual similarity to the target word?
(d) Does JT ever use a substitution and a target word in combination?
(e) Can an intervention from another speaker cue JT into producing the target word?
(f) Does JT ever follow a specific term by a semantically related general term?

6.5 Acquired aphasia 3

Background

Even in the presence of significant language impairment, adults with aphasia are often very resourceful in conveying their communicative intentions to listeners. A range of linguistic and non-linguistic strategies are used for this purpose. Prinz (1980) examined the ability of three adults with aphasia to make requests during conversations with an examiner. During 20-minute videotaped conversations, the examiner randomly introduced ten requesting elicitors. For example, the examiner might hand the subject a broken pencil and ask him to sign his name, prompting the subject to ask for another pencil. The requests produced by each of the three subjects, and the elicitors used, are shown below.

Elicitors

  (1) Offer patient a cigarette without a means to light it.
  (2) Talk about handwriting analysis. Give patient piece of paper with no writing utensil and ask him to sign his name.
  (3) Give patient a broken pencil and ask him to sign his name.
  (4) Give patient a pen. Mark three X's on the paper and ask him to sign next to the X without specifying which one.
  (5) Spill some coffee on the paper without offering to clean it up.
  (6) Offer patient something to drink without indicating what is available from the vending machines or cafeteria.
  (7) After going downstairs for something to drink, return with a large bandage (on experimenter's neck) without offering an explanation of what happened.
  (8) Start speaking a foreign language.
  (9) Show the patient a box which is locked.
(10) Show the patient some pictures of people unfamiliar to him.

Data 1: 59-year-old male with Broca's aphasia

Elicitor and request

  (1) One (Unin.) (gestures lighting a cigarette with a match).
  (2) Need (gestures writing).
  (3) No pencil pentil broke.
  (4) X 1, 2, (points to each X and looks up at experimenter after pointing to each one).
  (5) Oh no! (points to paper towels on another table and makes rubbing gestures).
  (6) Me having uh trites (interpreted as Sprite).
  (7) (Pointing) What you (Unin.).
  (8) (Puzzled expression) Huh? Kid me?
  (9) (Pointing to box) You open box?
(10) One who? (Pointing to each picture).

Data 2: 47-year-old male with Wernicke's aphasia

Elicitor and request

(1) Huh? No, I don't smoke. I don't want anything.
(2) Do you want Do you have something to write. Because I don't have anything to write (searches pockets).
(3) (Examines pencil) This one here-it's broken.
(4) Up here? Up here? (pointing to first X). Like this? Like that?
(5) Don't they-don't you have something that you (looking around room).
(6) No-something wet. Something to drink. Anything. (gestures drinking from a cup). You know-something to drink. I don't want coffee something cold.
(7) What'd you d-hurt yourself?
(8) I don't what is that?
(9) (Points) Yeh. What? Do you wanna open this?
(10) (Looks at pictures) I don't hear anything. Who is this? Who are these people?

Data 3: 37-year-old male with global aphasia

Elicitor and request

(1) (Points emphatically, smiles, leans forward) Mommy? (jargon, takes out his lighter).
(2) (Points to experimenter, looks in pocket, quizzical look) Pencil.
(3) (Shows broken end of pencil to experimenter and tries to whittle end of pencil with his fingernail).
(4) (Signs at first X without questioning which X).
(5) (Points to paper towels on next table).
(6) September no cold (with experimenter's assistance indicates lemonade).
(7) Mommy? (points to bandage, laughs, becomes serious).
(8) (Looks at experimenter, quizzical looks, laugh, waves arm as if to say 'forget it', points to paper and pen and then writes 'German').
(9) (Tries to open box).
(10) (Looks at pictures – returns them to experimenter as if to say, 'here you tell me who these people are'. – points to pictures one by one).

Exercise 1 Give two examples of each of the following errors in the above data sets:

(a) phonemic paraphasia
(b) semantic paraphasia

Exercise 2 Clearly, gesture plays an important role in the request strategies of these speakers. Give two examples of each of the following uses of gesture:

(a) Gestures take the place of spoken utterances.
(b) Gestures augment spoken utterances.
(c) Gestures are non-specific in nature and do not facilitate a request.
(d) Gestures are specific in nature and do facilitate a request.

Exercise 3 One of these speakers uses a stereotyped utterance when making requests. Which speaker is it and what is the utterance?

Exercise 4 Questions feature extensively in the request strategies of the subjects in Data 1 and Data 2. However, there is a significant difference between these subjects in the type of questions used. Indicate what this difference is and explain why it occurs.

Exercise 5 Beyond gestures and linguistic utterances, requests are also achieved by these speakers through other modes of communication. Using evidence to support your response, indicate three such modes.

6.5 Acquired aphasia 4

The following data are from several speakers with aphasia.

Speaker 1

Roy sustained a left-hemisphere cerebrovascular accident during waterskiing seven years previously. He is in his mid-to-late 40s at the time of data collection (Beeke et al., 2007).

um ... so s- er skiing ... er waterskiing ... yeh uh Greenbridge ... yeah? uh Kent ... uh ... uh ... four of them ... uuuhh ... blokes y'know ... uh ... uhhh ... boat ... and ... anyway ... sort of ... waterskiing ... and strange! ... sort of ... and then ... ur ... bang! [mimes falling over] ... funny ... and all of a sudden ... bang.

Speaker 2

This speaker (R) developed aphasia following a stroke in his early 40s. He is in conversation with a speech and language therapist (T) (Marshall, 2009).

T: Can you tell me how far you have got with selling your business R?
R: er ... Mr N (Mrs S: Your accountant).
R: Yes ... I've left it to him.
T: And how far has he got with it?
R: er ... one chap has come up with a er ... fee ... but there's three more coming.
T: That's quite good isn't it? Are they offers that you can accept?
R: Not really.
T: So you want slightly more?
R: Yes.
T: How quickly do you want to sell it?
R: As soon as possible ... just for me to ... call it a day ... but it could take as long as three months.
T: What will you do with the capital?
R: Put it into the ... one in the ... What's name ... bank.
T: What's happening to the staff?
R: er ... (waves) goodbye ... goodbye.

Speaker 3

Description of the cookie theft picture by a 61-year-old male with fluent jargon aphasia (Conroy et al., 2009). The cookie theft picture is from the Boston Diagnostic Aphasia

Examination (Goodglass et al., 2001). In the picture, a woman is standing at the kitchen sink drying a plate, while the sink is overflowing with water. Meanwhile, a boy (presumably, the woman's son) has climbed a stool which is rocking precariously and is taking cookies from a jar in the cupboard. A girl (presumably, the boy's sister) has her hand raised upwards to receive the cookies that her brother is taking.

She's filling the bowl of water. He's slipping off the [unintelligible utterance] on the ground, having to say, he's going to the ground. I think there's only two things to manage. He is, he is, she is going to . . . going to say 'surprise', look she is noticing.

Speaker 4

Description of the cookie theft picture (as above) by a 66-year-old male with fluent anomic aphasia (Conroy et al., 2009).

The woman is by the kitchen, stuff is running over onto the floor. She is . . . she cannot . . . the young fellow has got up to the cupboard and is about to fall off the seat. The young girl is after some from this lad.

Exercise 1 These speakers display word-finding problems. What features of their spoken output indicate that this is the case?

Exercise 2 Is there any evidence of circumlocution and semantic paraphasia in the verbal output of these speakers?

Exercise 3 What term is used to describe the verbal output of speaker 1? What aspects of language are retained and what aspects are omitted?

Exercise 4 Non-verbal communication is employed to good effect by two of these speakers. Which speakers use non-verbal communication to help convey their message? Which linguistic deficit is non-verbal communication effectively compensating?

Exercise 5 How would you characterize the receptive language skills and cognitive skills of speaker 2?

6.5 Acquired aphasia 5

The following data are from speakers with aphasia.

Extract 1

Exchange between a speech and language therapist (T) and an aphasic client called Martha (M) who was studied by Horton et al. (2004). The symbol (.) indicates a micro-pause.

T: (hands a picture of a loaf of bread to M) What's that then?
M: Oh yes that's my slice of /breuf/ (.) my slice of bread (hands picture to T).
T: Good (2.0) (hands a picture of a telephone to M) what about that one?
M: That's the /fin/ (.) the /fa/ (1.5) oh no.
T: Listen Martha (touches M on the hand) what's it for?
M: Oh for ringing (.) ringing Geraldine.

T: So you ring Geraldine on the . . .
M: Phone (.) oh yes the phone.
T: Brilliant.

Extract 2

AC is a 66-year-old right-handed male who was studied by Van Lancker Sidtis (2004). He suffered a left frontoparietal stroke which resulted in transcortical sensory aphasia. He produces fluent, well-articulated speech and repetition is intact. However, he has severely impaired comprehension and naming.

AC: I came, I saw, I conquered.
T: What else did you use to do? . . . Were you an engineer?
AC: Yes, I was an engineer. It's more important. It's that I . . . I said good morning. I said good morning. And . . . or . . . I didn't even say good morning. I just said Hi, how are you? How are you? And we . . . we . . . Hi, good morning. How are you. It was 9, 8:30, 9:00. I decided to . . . I did very, very well, and then, all of a sudden. It's a long story. But I think I know what I'm talking about. I hope so. I hope so, too.

Extract 3

Jef (J), a client examined by Dalemans et al. (2010), is describing to an interviewer (I) his experience of aphasia.

J: Yes, seeing those men there, there are a few that have a plate saying I have aphasia. I don't do that anymore . . . They don't give a shit, nothing! They don't call it out loud, they are very, how do I have to say it, euh, I euh, ohoh . . . (long silence).
I: Yes and how do you notice that, that they don't care?
J: Yes, yes, rapidly and much too much and to all to hectic and you can not keep track of it all.

Exercise 1 In Extract 1, what type of sound error does Martha make as she attempts to produce the word 'bread'?

Exercise 2 What type of cueing strategy does the therapist use in Extract 1 to encourage Martha to produce the target word 'phone'?

Exercise 3 The aphasic speaker in Extract 2 makes extensive use of a certain type of expression in his verbal output. What type of expression is this? Give three examples.

Exercise 4 What evidence is there in Extract 3 that Jef has a word-finding problem?

Exercise 5 How would you characterize Jef's verbal comprehension skills in Extract 3?

6.6 Right-hemisphere language disorder

Background

Speakers with right-hemisphere damage (RHD) experience language and communication problems which are quite unlike those found in clients with left-hemisphere damage (LHD). While speakers with LHD have impairments of structural language, most typically in the form of aphasia, clients with RHD often display intact structural language and marked deficits in pragmatic and discourse skills.

Data

The following extract is taken from Abusamra et al. (2009: 77–8). It is a dialogue between an examiner (E) and a male patient (P) with RHD. The patient has been asked to explain the meaning of one of the metaphors from the MEC protocol (Joanette et al., 2004).

E: What does this phrase mean: My friend's mother-in-law is a witch?
P: Let's change also one word: My son-in-law's mother-in-law is a witch?
E: And so what does it mean?
P: I know she is a person who hasn't had a pleasant life, throughout her marriage. That . . . that she's about to be separated from her husband; I'm referring to the mother-in-law of my son-in-law (ha, ha, ha).
E: OK it's not important – it's the same.
P: Certainly! The mother-in-law of my son-in-law. The mother-in-law of my son-in-law is a witch!
E: What does being a witch mean?
P: Because the woman is separated, because all her life she has criticized her husband for the way he is; only seen in his defects, who has kept his daughter all her life under a glass bell and she's now a poor lady because she can't find the fiancé her mother would like.
E: So what does witch mean, then?
P: What does it specifically mean? It means being tied down to religious sects, to religions, to umbanda . . . who knows, there are so many.
E: So therefore, 'The mother-in-law of my son-in-law is a witch'. Does it mean the mother-in-law of my friend practices black magic? And the mother-in-law of my friend has many brooms and she is also a bad person and rude?
P: It's absolutely clear. My friend's mother-in-law has many brooms . . . no! My friend's mother-in-law practices black magic.

Exercise 1 Humour is an important aspect of pragmatic language use. Does this client make appropriate use of humour in his exchange with the examiner? Use data from the exchange to support your answer.

Exercise 2 Clients with right-hemisphere language disorder often produce egocentric discourse. Is there any evidence of this in the above exchange?

Exercise 3 How would you characterize P's understanding of the metaphor presented to him? Use data from the exchange to support your answer.

Exercise 4 Does P display any awareness that his interpretation of the examiner's metaphor may not be accurate?

Exercise 5 How would you characterize P's use of referring expressions? Use data from the exchange to support your answer.

6.7   Traumatic brain injury

Background

The following narratives were produced by two adults with traumatic brain injury who were studied by Biddle et al. (1996). Both adults were within 12 months of their injury at the time of interview. They were asked to recount an occasion on which they had got lost.

Data 1: 31-year-old man with TBI

(Long pause) About the only really good time I can remember getting lost was in West Virginia. Me and my brother had been walking into the woods one day and we found a pig in the woods. A pig. Pig got out of my uncle's . . . pig, uh . . . So we found a pig around. And then we found out that we did get lost. So we went walking through the woods for about two hours, until it got really dark. Then we found a house and went back home. But during the time that we were lost, we were really scared cause we didn't think we were going to make it back. And I got all upset and started crying like a little wimp. And I didn't think we were goin make it back. But we did. It was a little traumatic for me . . . cause I didn't think we were going to make it.

Data 2: 41-year-old woman with TBI

Well, I've gotten lost even coming here. It was probably the second time I came here. I, uh, went down, uh, 27, no 96, I think. And I came up . . . I remember they said 14 mile. I thought ended. Well, anyways, I just went around and around in circles. And uh . . . so I got lost there. And it doesn't seem . . . I do drive myself when I come here but I still get confused. I don't get lost but I get scared. I see Southfield Road and then I just . . . Southfield and Greenfield. And still, after coming since February, I'm still not sure whether for a few minutes, a few seconds there if I'm supposed to take Greenfield or Southfield, you know. And then I don't know Southfield, you know. And, uh . . . I did get lost the second time I came here.

Exercise 1 In Data 1, the speaker places a considerable burden on his listener through the provision of incomplete information. On one occasion in particular, the listener must make a number of inferences in order to connect two events. Identify the occasion in question and suggest what inferences the listener may need to draw.

Exercise 2 The speaker in Data 1 produces some repetitive language. Identify where this occurs in the extract.

Exercise 3 A number of discourse and linguistic anomalies occur in Data 2. Provide <u>one</u> example of each of the following anomalies in the extract:

(a) The narrative contains repetitive language.
(b) The speaker begins utterances only to abandon them.
(c) The speaker omits necessary grammatical parts.
(d) The speaker displays referential disturbances.
(e) The speaker conveys contradictory information.

Exercise 4 Give <u>two</u> possible explanations of the speaker's use of filled pauses in data 2.

Exercise 5 Is discourse cohesion used appropriately by both speakers? Present data to support your answer.

6.8   Dementias 1

Background

The following extracts of data have been produced by adults with Alzheimer's dementia (Chapman et al., 1998). The data were collected during a range of discourse production tasks. The tasks involved (a) retelling fables, (b) capturing the gist of fables, (c) conveying the lesson of fables, (d) story generation based on a single frame picture, and (e) verbal explanations of the meaning of proverbs. Each of these tasks places different demands on a speaker's cognitive, linguistic and pragmatic skills. Examine each extract and then answer the questions below.

Fable retelling

Subjects read and heard the following fable, which they were then required to retell:

A hungry raven saw that pigeons in the pigeon coop had a lot of food. He painted his feathers white to look like them. But when he started to crow, they realized that he was a raven and chased him away. So he returned to his own kind. But the other ravens did not recognize him because he had his feathers painted white, so they also chased him away.

Extract 1: Uh, you know, the raven uh, like any-any bird has got to eat, and the way they get their food is uh, apparently by guile. By uh, uh, confusing the uh, other . . . whatever the hell it was. I forgot. Um, it was a raven and what else? (Examiner: The raven and the pigeon.) Pigeon, okay. Uh, the raven uh-uh, was gonna do whatever he's needed to do to accomplish the goal uh, which was to get some food uh, when this uh, rabbit had plenty of food and he didn't, so he uh-uh, used his head and figured the program out and uh . . . achieved the end that he was after, the more food.

Gist of fables

Subjects were required to capture the main idea or gist of a fable.

Extract 2: Uh, well, just the main idea is that uh, any animal or person or anything else will do whatever they have to do to get the food they need to survive. Survival of the fittest, I guess.

Lesson of fables

Subjects were asked to convey a lesson which could be learned from a fable.

Extract 3: Uh . . . I guess work hard and persevere and you won't have to uh, steal your food.

Story generation

Subjects were shown a single-frame, contextually rich picture. They were asked to observe the picture, and generate a story based on it. The story was related to the examiner while the picture was face down. The picture was a Norman Rockwell print which depicted a rural scene around the 1930s. The picture displays an older man dressed in work clothes who is smoking a rolled cigarette. There is a young man dressed in a suit. He has a small wrapped parcel, books and a suitcase, the latter with a State U. sticker on it. There is also a sheep dog with his head on the young man's lap. Both men are sitting next to each other on the running board of an old truck.

Extract 4: Well, uh there is a man there and there is uh looks like a child and um there's a dog and I think there's an older man there too. I think so. Um I think that's an older man in the picture. Um it looks it's an autumn day out there and it's kind of overcast, kinda like it is today. Um, and the man and the boy are talking and uh I think that the boy, the little guy, I think that they are going fishing or they're thinking about going fishing.

Proverb meaning

Subjects were asked to explain the meaning of the proverb 'One swallow doesn't make a summer'.

Extract 5: Um . . . one swallow doesn't make a summer. Mmmm, I don't know what to say to that. Uh (5 seconds) Oh, we're not talking about the swallow as a bird, are we? One swallow doesn't make a summer. Umm . . . one swallow doesn't make a summer- one swallow- one bird doesn't make a . . . one, more than one way to skin a cat, is it? Um . . . well, just because someone is doing this job, doing it that way doesn't mean you can't do it a different way and uh, and reach the same conclusion.

Exercise 1 The speaker in Extract 1 displays relatively good expressive language skills. However, there is evidence of a particular linguistic difficulty. What is that difficulty and how is it manifested in the extract?

Exercise 2 Extracts 2 and 3 are unsatisfactory attempts at capturing the gist and lesson of fables, respectively. In what respect are they unsatisfactory?

Exercise 3 In Extract 4, is the subject generating a story or merely describing a picture? Present linguistic evidence to support your decision.

Exercise 4 Extract 5 is not satisfactory as an explanation of the meaning of the proverb presented to the subject. Explain why it is unsatisfactory.

Exercise 5 Which of the following statements best captures these extracts?

(a) The extracts are verbose.
(b) The extracts are over-informative.
(c) The extracts exhibit considerable tangentiality.
(d) The extracts convey information in an appropriate amount of language.
(e) The extracts are markedly under-informative.

6.8   Dementias 2

Background

The following extracts are from adult patients with fluent and non-fluent primary progressive aphasia (PPA) and frontal lobe dementia (FLD) who were studied by Orange et al. (1998).

Extract 1: Subject BV (65-year-old female) with non-fluent PPA; Examiner (E), Subject (S)

E: And your address?
S: Um it's uh R or . . .
S: No wait a minute!
S: It's um . . .
S: That's not right um today.
S: It it's in Clinton.
E: Uhhuh.
S: And and um it's uh four no . . .
S: Oh dear.
S: Um let's see.
S: Clinton and um . . .
S: Oh gosh.
S: My uh address is um ah . . .
S: Oh gosh.

Extract 2: Subject RH (78-year-old female) with non-fluent PPA

E: Tell me your full name.
S: R G H (full name spoken).
S: And I don't very much very very much about uh um um day.
S: And my uh my father's dead.
S: My father uh you know he was really . . .
S: We'd he's awful.

Extract 3: Subject EB (65-year-old male) with FLD

E: What problems have you been having Mr B?
S: Uh I had an M I R (spelled each letter) and and a and and I had a C A T scan (spelled).
S: And I proper proper name is and the and it's called . . .
E: But those are the tests that you've had.
E: What is your problem?

Extract 4: Subject VB (75-year-old female) with fluent PPA

E: Have you been here before?
S: Where?
E: In this hospital?
S: For mmh something that happen to me?
E: Uhhuh.
S: No.
S: Yesterday in with professor or doctor oh . . .
S: Damn.
S: I am thinking of his name.
S: It's coming but uh . . .
S: When I when I am tense everything goes (gestures with hands).

Exercise 1 One of these subjects makes extensive use of stereotyped utterances and incomplete utterances. Which subject is it? Give <u>two</u> examples of each type of utterance. What do these utterances reveal about this subject's language skills?

Exercise 2 Problems with topic relevance are evident in the above data. Which subjects display these problems? Describe the problems these subjects have with topic relevance.

Exercise 3 One of these subjects displays awareness of his or her language problems. Which subject is it? What type of language impairment is this subject describing?

Exercise 4 Which two language levels are most impaired in these subjects? Provide evidence for your answer.

Exercise 5 Why is an assessment of syntax difficult in the subjects in Extracts 1 and 2?

6.8 Dementias 3

Background

Warren is a 36-year-old right-handed man who was studied by McCabe et al. (2008). He has a mixed employment history that includes work as a nursing assistant, personal carer, short-order cook, housekeeper and various handyman positions. He ceased work in the 12 months preceding the initial assessment due to peripheral neuropathy and AIDS dementia complex (ADC). He had completed 13 years of education including a general nurses' aide certificate. He frequently spoke of returning to the workforce and of completing a degree in occupational therapy.

Warren lives alone and acquired HIV from male-to-male sexual activity. He has had a number of opportunistic infections including oral and anal candida (thrush), pneumonia and systemic cytomegalovirus infection. He had previously been prescribed various combinations of antiviral drugs but had self-reported poor compliance with these treatment regimes. Warren has been diagnosed with ADC by an AIDS specializing neurologist. Before diagnosis of dementia there was no history of cognitive-learning or language impairment, psychiatric illness, or any neurological impairment and Warren has no family history of speech or language impairment. Warren reported no changes in his communication skills since HIV infection.

Data: Warren (W), Examiner (E)

E: What would be the longest job you had?
W: Oh, when I had the business, cleaning the building
E: Mm and that was for how many years?
W: Eight years, like I said I was spoiled
E: And that was when you were in your twenties?
W: Twenty two. (Name) was the only person who had total faith in me. There was an intelligent person in there that, um, he said I've got more common sense. I like that idea 'cause there's nothing common about this little black duck and if I am on my way to prove that I'm not. My great grandmother was born into a family that was indentured to a castle near Salisbury, Newcastle. Well she was supposed to be a house servant. She sort of looked at then at the age

of 17 and said 'Do I look like a peasant girl to you? I don't think so, I'm jumping on a boat and going to Australia . . . ' (continued in same vein for six more utterances).

Exercise 1 Does Warren display any problems with the use of syntax? If so, what are these problems?

Exercise 2 Is there evidence of a word-finding deficit in Warren's verbal output? Does Warren display an impairment of auditory comprehension?

Exercise 3 How would you characterize Warren's management of topic in this exchange?

Exercise 4 Does Warren develop meaning associations between utterances? What other clinical group displays this linguistic behaviour?

Exercise 5 How would you characterize Warren's use of referencing in this exchange?

SUGGESTIONS FOR FURTHER READING

Bastiaanse, R. and Prins, R. S. 2014. 'Aphasia', in L. Cummings (ed.), *Cambridge handbook of communication disorders*, Cambridge: Cambridge University Press, 224–46.

Cummings, L. 2008. *Clinical linguistics*, Edinburgh: Edinburgh University Press (section 5.4).
    2014a. *Communication disorders*, Houndmills: Palgrave Macmillan (chapter 5).

Joanette, Y., Ferré, P. and Wilson, M. A. 2014. 'Right hemisphere damage and communication', in L. Cummings (ed.), *Cambridge handbook of communication disorders*, Cambridge: Cambridge University Press, 247–65.

Le, K., Mozeiko, J. and Coelho, C. 2010. 'Traumatic brain injury and discourse', in L. Cummings (ed.), *Routledge pragmatics encyclopedia*, London and New York: Routledge, 475–8.

Maxim, J. and Bryan, K. 2006. 'Language, communication and cognition in the dementias', in K. Bryan and J. Maxim (eds.), *Communication disability in the dementias*, Chichester: Whurr, 73–124.

Monetta, L. and Champagne-Lavau, M. 2010. 'Right-hemisphere damage and pragmatics', in L. Cummings (ed.), *Routledge pragmatics encyclopedia*, London and New York: Routledge, 408–9.

Orange, J. B. and Williams, L. J. 2010. 'Dementia and conversation', in L. Cummings (ed.), *Routledge pragmatics encyclopedia*, London and New York: Routledge, 105–8.

Reilly, J. and Hung, J. 2014. 'Dementia and communication', in L. Cummings (ed.), *Cambridge handbook of communication disorders*, Cambridge: Cambridge University Press, 266–83.

Togher, L. 2014. 'Traumatic brain injury and communication', in L. Cummings (ed.), *Cambridge handbook of communication disorders*, Cambridge: Cambridge University Press, 284–99.

Chapter 7

Disorders of voice

A significant number of children and adults experience problems with the production of voice or phonation which compromise their effectiveness as communicators. Many voice disorders or dysphonias have an identifiable organic aetiology. This may take the form of benign growths known as vocal nodules, which are related to sustained vocal abuse. Unsurprisingly, vocal nodules are commonly found in children who regularly shout and scream and in professional voice users (e.g. singers) who place above average demands on their voice. Alternatively, a malignant growth may pervade the tissues of the larynx to such an extent that a partial or complete laryngectomy is necessitated. The adult who undergoes a laryngectomy can achieve voice production after surgery through the use of an artificial or electronic larynx, the production of oesophageal voice or surgical voice reconstruction. Aside from benign and malignant growths, other organic aetiologies of voice disorders include infections (e.g. viral laryngitis), neurological impairment (e.g. vocal fold paralysis), vocal fold haemorrhage, and laryngeal trauma (e.g. as a result of endotracheal intubation). Speech and language therapists work closely with ENT specialists (or otolaryngologists) in the assessment and treatment of organic voice disorders.

In a significant number of clients, voice disorders occur in the absence of an identifiable organic aetiology. So-called functional or psychogenic voice disorders include conditions such as puberphonia (primarily in adolescent males) and conversion aphonia which can arise in response to a significant psychological trauma. Owing to the presence of psychological factors in the development and maintenance of functional voice disorders, speech and language therapists often work closely with clinical psychologists and psychiatrists in the assessment and treatment of these dysphonias. In reality, however, most voice disorders have organic and psychological components. For example, an adult may routinely engage in hyperadduction of the vocal folds in response to various psychological stressors. However, this pattern of voice use may damage the vocal fold mucosa and lead ultimately to the development of vocal nodules. In this case, the client's voice disorder has clear psychological and organic components within its aetiology.

Clients who undergo gender reassignment surgery have specific communication needs which are assessed and treated by speech and language therapists. Post-operative voice production, especially in the male-to-female transsexual, is an area of particular concern.

Section A: Short-answer questions

7.1 Organic voice disorders

(1) Fill in the blank spaces in these paragraphs using the words in the box below:
Organic voice disorders can affect all age groups. The premature baby may require intensive medical intervention in the first days and weeks of its life. Prolonged _____ in the premature infant can cause unilateral vocal fold paralysis. Several chromosomal and genetic _____ involve structural abnormalities of the larynx. For example,

abnormalities such as laryngeal hypoplasia are responsible for the distinctive cat-like cry in _____ syndrome. In children, recurrent respiratory _____ is the most common benign neoplasm of the airway. The disease frequently involves the larynx. Other benign growths that are found on the vocal folds of children are _____ . These growths develop in the child who is engaged in repeated _____ of his vocal mechanism (e.g. shouting at friends in the playground at school).

Adults who drink and smoke heavily are at risk of developing a malignant _____ of the larynx. In the case of advanced tumours, a _____ must be performed. Post-operatively, the laryngectomee may be taught to communicate using an _____ larynx, _____ speech or _____ restoration (e.g. the use of a Blom-Singer valve). Finally, the larynx can deteriorate with advancing years leading to a voice disorder called _____ . These age-related changes include vocal fold bowing and atrophy.

glossectomy	syndromes	abuse	tumour
presbylarynx	muscle tension dysphonia		nodules
intubation	cri du chat	artificial/electronic	
cricothyroid approximation	laryngectomy		
papillomatosis	surgical voice	oesophageal	

(2) Which of the following are *true* statements about organic voice disorders?
   (a) Laryngeal tuberculosis can cause voice disorder.
   (b) Vocal intensity increases in individuals with Parkinson's disease.
   (c) Drugs such as aspirin can cause vocal fold haemorrhages.
   (d) Hormonal changes associated with menstruation and the menopause can alter voice quality in women.
   (e) Bilateral vocal fold paralysis can compromise a person's airway and may require a laryngectomy to be performed.

(3) Which of the following is *not* a cause of an organic voice disorder?
   (a) infectious disease
   (b) neurological disorder
   (c) conversion disorder
   (d) congenital defect
   (e) vocal abuse and misuse

(4) Which of the following statements is *not* true of laryngeal papillomas?
   (a) Laryngeal papillomas are caused by human papilloma virus types 6 and 22.
   (b) Laryngeal papillomas grow quickly and can recur after surgical removal.
   (c) Laryngeal papillomas can compromise the airway.
   (d) Laryngeal papillomas may cause stridor.
   (e) Laryngeal papillomas are benign growths.

(5) In which of the following conditions does vocal fold bowing occur?
   (a) presbylarynx
   (b) Reinke's oedema
   (c) vocal fold haemorrhage
   (d) inadequate innervation of the vocal folds
   (e) spasmodic dysphonia

(6) Which of the following is *not* associated with vocal fold paralysis and paresis (VFPP)?
  (a) VFPP always necessitates a tracheotomy.
  (b) There may be no known cause for VFPP.
  (c) VFPP may result from damage to the recurrent laryngeal nerve and/or the superior laryngeal nerve.
  (d) Bilateral VFPP compromises the airway.
  (e) VFPP can cause stridor.

(7) Aetiologies which are not structural or neurological in nature can also cause organic voice disorders. Which of the following constitutes such an aetiology?
  (a) hyperthyroidism
  (b) granulomas
  (c) inhaled corticosteroids
  (d) tuberculosis
  (e) laryngeal trauma

(8) Which of the following statements is *not* true of vocal nodules and polyps?
  (a) Vocal nodules and polyps are benign growths.
  (b) Vocal nodules tend to be larger than polyps.
  (c) Vocal nodules and polyps develop at the middle of the vocal folds.
  (d) Vocal nodules are seldom found on both vocal folds.
  (e) Vocal nodules tend to be more common in certain occupational groups (e.g. teachers).

(9) Complete the blank spaces in the following statements:
  (a) During thoracic surgery, the _____ nerve may be damaged, leading to a voice disorder.
  (b) A mucous-retention cyst has _____ content and is caused by the obstruction of _____ ducts.
  (c) The presence of a cyst causes the vocal fold to bulge or protrude. By repeatedly making contact with the other vocal fold, the protruding fold can cause a _____ to develop in it.
  (d) Granulomas are a benign inflammatory lesion of the vocal folds. They are most often located over the vocal process of the _____ cartilage.
  (e) Vocal folds may bleed or haemorrhage causing tiny, visible capillaries called _____ or capillary ectasias.

(10) For each of the following statements indicate if it is *True* or *False*:
  (a) There is an increased prevalence of voice disorder in subjects with rheumatoid arthritis.
  (b) Polypoid inflammation is another term for Reinke's oedema.
  (c) Glottal leakage can occur in sulcus vocalis, resulting in a breathy voice.
  (d) In adductor spasmodic dysphonia, the vocal folds fail to maintain normal contact during phonation.
  (e) Spasmodic dysphonia is a common voice disorder in the professional voice user.

7.2 Functional voice disorders

(1) *True* or *False*: Conversion aphonia is a voice disorder of organic aetiology.

(2) *True* or *False*: A voice disorder related to the presence of benign growths on the vocal folds is functional in nature.

(3) *True* or *False*: Hyperfunctional dysphonias involve excessive laryngeal and supralaryngeal tension.

(4) A professional voice user presents at a voice clinic with severe hoarseness. Examination reveals severe reddening of the laryngeal mucosa. Further investigation reveals that this is caused by gastroesophageal reflux. This individual's voice disorder has:
(a) an organic aetiology only
(b) a functional aetiology only
(c) an organic and functional aetiology
(d) a psychogenic aetiology
(e) none of the above

(5) Which of the following is *not* associated with conversion aphonia?
(a) Loss of voice occurs in response to a traumatic event or some other psychological stressor.
(b) Conversion aphonia is more commonly found in males than in females.
(c) Colds and flues and associated laryngitis can serve as a trigger.
(d) Vocal folds adduct normally during vegetative phonation (e.g. coughing).
(e) Treatment often involves psychological therapy alongside speech and language therapy.

(6) During adolescence, some males resist the voice _____ that occurs in their peers. These males continue to speak with a pre-pubescent voice. This condition is called _____.

(7) _____ voice users (e.g. singers) can develop voice problems. Vocal abuse and misuse certainly contribute to the development of voice difficulties in this group. However, _____ factors such as anxiety also play a role in abuse-related dysphonias.

(8) *True* or *False*: In muscle tension dysphonia, approximation of the false vocal folds is one of the laryngeal findings.

(9) Which of the following statements characterize assessment of the voice client by the speech and language therapist (SLT)?
(a) The SLT performs a perceptual evaluation of the voice.
(b) The SLT performs an instrumental assessment of the voice.
(c) The SLT works closely with a range of medical professionals (e.g. otolaryngologist, gastroenterologist, neurologist) in assessing voice disorders in clients.
(d) The SLT uses electropalatography to assess voice disorders.
(e) The SLT performs a neurological evaluation of the voice client.

(10) Which of the following statements characterize treatment of the voice client by the speech and language therapist (SLT)?
(a) The SLT is primarily responsible for the treatment of voice disorders that are related to gastroesophageal reflux.
(b) The SLT advises the client with abuse-related dysphonia on techniques of safe voice use.
(c) The SLT gives advice to clients on the detrimental effects of environmental agents (e.g. smoke) on the vocal mechanism.
(d) The SLT often works closely with psychotherapists and counsellors in the treatment of voice disorders.
(e) The SLT has a negligible role to play in the treatment of voice in transsexual clients.

7.3 Laryngectomy

(1) Which of the following statements is *not* associated with laryngectomy?

    (a) The patient breathes through a neck stoma.

    (b) An electronic or artificial larynx is only used in the days and weeks following surgery and is gradually phased out during post-operative speech and language therapy.

    (c) The cricopharyngeus muscle in the oesophagus is integral to the production of oesophageal voice.

    (d) A speaking valve directs the pulmonary airstream into the neck stoma.

    (e) Techniques of non-laryngeal voice production may be combined (e.g. electronic larynx and oesophageal voice).

(2) *True* or *False*: Surgical voice restoration is playing an increasingly important role in the management of clients who undergo laryngectomy.

(3) Fill in the blank spaces in these paragraphs using the words in the box below:

Malignant growths of the larynx are less _____ than benign lesions. However, these growths are ultimately more destructive of the larynx and its surrounding tissues than benign lesions. The large majority of laryngeal cancers are _____ carcinomas, although several other types of malignancies can also occur. A chondrosarcoma is a rare tumour that affects the _____ of the larynx. When a malignant tumour is diagnosed by the otolaryngologist, intervention involving a combination of _____ and surgery is usually indicated. Depending on the extent of a tumour, a _____ or a total laryngectomy may be undertaken. The removal of the larynx during _____ necessitates the establishment of an alternative route for respiration. The surgeon must direct the trachea onto the patient's neck, where a permanent tracheal _____ will be formed for _____ and expectoration. Where a laryngeal tumour is advanced, further surgical procedures may be required, including _____ dissection, pharyngolaryngectomy and pharyngo-laryngo-oesophagectomy. The last two procedures are necessary when there is extensive involvement of the _____ and oesophagus.

Surgery is now also playing an increasing role in restoring _____ to the laryngectomy client. A tracheoesophageal voice _____ provides a route for pulmonary air to enter the oesophagus, where it vibrates the pharyngo-oesophageal segment. The airstream is directed from the _____ into the oesophagus by means of the manual occlusion of the stoma or, alternatively, the use of a _____ valve. The resulting voice is more easily produced than _____ voice. It is also of higher _____ and greater fluency than oesophageal voice. Although surgical voice _____ is increasingly being performed at the same time as laryngectomy, it has not completely replaced other forms of voice production. Clients continue to use an artificial or _____ larynx following laryngectomy as either their only means of non-laryngeal voice production or in combination with other methods (e.g. oesophageal voice).

pharyngeal	respiration	voice	pitch	cartilage
tracheostoma	basal cell	partial	restoration	common
squamous cell	oesophageal	tongue	stoma	trachea
intensity	pharynx	glossectomy	electronic	laryngectomy
chemotherapy	neck	palate	prosthesis	radiotherapy

(4) *True* or *False*: Following laryngectomy, a patient's stoma may become infected and may close over.

(5) *True* or *False*: The client who undergoes a laryngectomy may experience dysphagia after surgery.

(6) *True* or *False*: Oesophageal voice production is only pursued as a form of communication after all other methods have failed.

(7) Which of the following statements describes the role of the speech and language therapist (SLT) in the management of the client who undergoes a laryngectomy?
   (a) The SLT diagnoses a malignant laryngeal carcinoma and recommends a partial or a total laryngectomy.
   (b) The SLT advises nursing staff on the post-operative medical care of the client.
   (c) The SLT meets the client pre-operatively to discuss the implications of surgery for voice production.
   (d) The SLT decides pre-operatively on a form of non-laryngeal voice production for the client.
   (e) The SLT discusses all forms of non-laryngeal voice production with the client both pre- and post-operatively.

(8) Which of the following factors has been linked to the development of laryngeal carcinoma?
   (a) gastroesophageal reflux disease
   (b) immunosuppression
   (c) inhaled corticosteroids
   (d) consumption of caffeinated drinks
   (e) human papillomavirus 16

(9) If a nerve supplying the tongue is severed during laryngectomy, the _____ of speech sounds is likely to be compromised.

(10) Recurrent advanced-stage laryngeal cancers are generally treated by _____ laryngectomy.

7.4   Gender dysphoria

(1) Which of the following is *not* one of the diagnostic criteria for gender identity disorder?
   (a) A physical intersex condition should be present.
   (b) A strong and persistent cross-gender identification should be present.
   (c) A persistent discomfort with the gender role of one's sex should be present.
   (d) Impairment in social or occupational functioning should be present.
   (e) An individual should not have Turner's syndrome.

(2) *True* or *False*: Gender identity disorder is more commonly found in females than in males.

(3) Which of the following areas is the focus of speech and language therapy with the transsexual client?
   (a) articulation
   (b) pragmatics
   (c) intensity of speaking voice

(d) pitch of speaking voice

(e) expressive syntax

(4) Long-term changes in _____ frequency can be achieved through voice therapy with the transsexual client, although these changes do not always result in alterations in listener perceptions of gender.

(5) In cricothyroid approximation, the cricoid cartilage and _____ are approximated and held in position by sutures.

(6) Phonosurgery is more often pursued by the male-to-female (MTF) transsexual than by the female-to-male (FTM) transsexual because:
   (a) Removal of the testes and oestrogen therapy in the MTF transsexual may achieve only minor changes in the pitch of the voice.
   (b) Surgical changes to the larynx are more difficult to bring about in the FTM transsexual.
   (c) FTM transsexuals are in general less concerned about the pitch of their voice than MTF transsexuals.
   (d) Androgen therapy is generally successful in achieving desired pitch changes in FTM transsexuals without the need for surgical intervention.
   (e) FTM transsexuals are less inclined to pursue phonosurgery because they undergo more major surgery than MTF transsexuals during gender reassignment surgery.

(7) Which of the following statements characterize the role of the speech and language therapist (SLT) in the management of the transsexual client?
   (a) The SLT's role is to instruct the client in how to avoid damaging patterns of voice use.
   (b) The SLT's role is to recommend a hormonal treatment that will achieve desired pitch changes of the voice.
   (c) The SLT's role is to recommend the type of phonosurgery that is most suitable for the client.
   (d) The SLT's role is to employ conventional voice therapy techniques in an attempt to alter the pitch of the client's voice.
   (e) The SLT's role is to counsel the client on the occupational and social implications of gender reassignment surgery.

(8) *True* or *False*: Voice alterations in the transsexual client can only be effectively achieved through hormone treatments.

(9) *True* or *False*: A diagnosis of gender identity disorder is made on the basis of criteria that are set out in the Diagnostic and Statistical Manual of Mental Disorders.

(10) *True* or *False*: Voice surgery should always be recommended to the transsexual client as the primary method of achieving desired vocal changes.

Section B: Data analysis exercises

7.5   Organic voice disorders

Background

Both of the case studies presented below involve organic voice disorders. Examine the details of these cases and then answer the questions which follow.

Case A

NB, a 61-year-old Caucasian female, complained of irregular speech breaks without hoarseness or aphonia. Symptoms started about two years ago. The patient underwent assessment by means of stroboscopy, clinical neurological exam and voice lab. She presented signs of tense voice, vocal tiredness, breathy voice, laryngeal pain, loss of voice extension and lack of frequency control. Stroboscopy revealed mild bilateral vocal tremor which was more intense in the left vocal fold. There were no structural lesions on the vocal folds and no oedema. NB had good lamina propria expansion bilaterally without glottal gaps. She was treated with the injection of Botulin toxin (Botox) in the left thyroarytenoid muscle. Her voice was somewhat breathy in the first week and after that it became stable (Santos et al., 2006: 426).

Case B

NAR, a 44-year-old female, complained of hoarseness, vocal tiredness and weak voice since childhood. She did not smoke and did not complain of reflux. Her voice sounded high, blowy, with vocal effort and reduction in phonation time. Laryngological examination revealed a spindle-like cleft. The patient refused to undergo surgery. Her case history revealed that she had three brothers with dysphonia. These brothers were aged 22, 29 and 42. Two reported hoarseness and weak voice since childhood. The third brother reported mild hoarseness during vocal abuse. All three brothers denied smoking and experienced vocal symptoms similar to NAR. One brother had undergone phonosurgery in the form of a fat graft (Martins et al., 2007: 573).

Exercise 1 In one of the above cases, the laryngeal pathology is structural in nature. Identify this case and the laryngeal pathology involved. Which factors were significant in your choice of disorder?

Exercise 2 In one of the above cases, the laryngeal pathology is neurological in nature. Identify this case and the laryngeal pathology involved. Which factors were significant in your choice of disorder?

Exercise 3 Which of the following statements best describes stroboscopy?

(a) Stroboscopy is an instrumental assessment technique which permits clinicians to observe velopharyngeal valving.
(b) Stroboscopy enables the otolaryngologist to observe vocal fold vibratory function during phonation.
(c) Stroboscopy assesses a client's ability to coordinate the phonatory and respiratory systems during speech production.
(d) Stroboscopy provides measurements of the vegetative functions of the larynx.
(e) Stroboscopy is never performed alongside other instrumental assessments.

Exercise 4 Apart from the laryngeal pathology you identified for case B, name one other organic voice disorder which a fat graft may be used to treat.

Exercise 5 Which of the following are *true* statements about the lamina propria?

(a) The lamina propria is a thin layer of stratified squamous epithelium which covers the vocal folds.
(b) The lamina propria consists of superficial, intermediate and deep layers.
(c) The three layers of the lamina propria together comprise the mucosa of the vocal fold.
(d) The lamina propria is a pliable layer of fibrous proteins which account for its unique biomechanical properties.
(e) The lamina propria is a laryngeal cartilage.

7.6 Functional voice disorders

Background

Both of the case studies presented below involve functional voice disorders. Examine the details of these cases and then answer the questions which follow.

Case A

Judith, a 53-year-old professional woman, first experienced hoarseness and voice loss two months prior to her voice evaluation. She reported a sudden onset to her voice problems, intermittent pitch breaks and frequent coughing. It was difficult for Judith to project her voice or sing. She described a feeling of fullness in her throat and of food sticking in her throat. Her professional and personal life was being adversely affected by her voice problems. Judith reported having an anxiety disorder and occasionally had panic attacks. She does not smoke or drink alcohol. During the week she works long hours and she volunteers with several organizations at the weekend.

A diagnosis of laryngopharyngeal reflux was made following flexible nasendoscopy. Reflux symptoms are reported to have improved since Judith starting taking medication some three weeks before her voice evaluation. Laryngeal findings included oedema and erythema (redness) of the arytenoid cartilages and cartilaginous portion of the vocal folds along with tissue hypertrophy of the posterior glottis. There was no evidence of contact ulcers or granulomas. Medial compression of the vocal folds with a large posterior glottal chink was revealed by stroboscopy. There were thick mucous strands across the vocal folds and the mucosal wave was reduced.

Judith's voice evaluation revealed anomalies in pitch, quality and respiration. Her speaking fundamental frequency in contextual speech (174 Hz) was low for her age and gender. Judith's fundamental frequency pitch range (133–348 Hz) was not within normal limits. A frequency perturbation of 2.85 for /a/ correlated perceptually to vocal hoarseness. She displayed moderate to severe breathiness, mild to moderate roughness and moderate strain. Breaks in phonation and hard glottal attack upon initiation of phonation were heard. The maximum phonation duration for sustained /a/ was 9 seconds, which is not within normal limits for Judith's age and gender. Judith displayed a number of vocal abuse behaviours including coughing, talking excessively, throat clearing and singing (Gallena, 2007: 24–5).

Case B

AB, a 23-year-old female student, experienced viral laryngitis with subsequent loss of voice and a whispery dysphonia for three weeks. She underwent otolaryngological examination which revealed muscle tension dysphonia, anteroposterior constriction and normal vocal fold movement on coughing. There was no other laryngeal pathology. AB was told that her dysphonia was related to laryngitis and protective tension of the laryngeal muscles. She was referred to speech pathology to work on correct use of the voice.

A full psychosocial interview was conducted at AB's first speech pathology session, which she attended with her mother. Normal phonation was readily elicited during coughing and facilitating exercises and this was quickly consolidated into comfortable conversational speech. Psychogenic dysphonia was explained to AB and her mother with the therapist discussing physical, functional and psychosocial or emotional influences on the voice as part of her explanation. AB explored these potential factors with the therapist and her mother and felt that her ongoing studies and work pressure were the only factors that might be of significance in the development of her voice disorder. However, AB still believed these could not fully account for her voice problems and wondered if there might be an alternative explanation. Although AB left the session happy with the outcome, the therapist felt that the problem had not been fully resolved.

At her second session a week later, which she attended on her own, AB appeared relaxed and chatted at ease about her studies and work. It was towards the end of the session when AB quietly asked the therapist if an event some four months earlier could have given rise to her voice problems. She recounted how she had been brutally raped by a young man on her course, who had taken her to his family home. She tried to scream during the assault, but was unable to make anyone in the house hear her. AB did not report the assault for fear of academic and career repercussions. The man responsible for the attack had been assigned to AB's immediate work environment at the beginning of the week in which AB had developed viral laryngitis and subsequent dysphonia (Baker, 2003: 311–12).

Exercise 1 In one of the above cases, the functional voice disorder is psychogenic in nature. Identify this case and the voice disorder involved. Which factors were significant in your choice of disorder?

Exercise 2 In one of the above cases, the functional voice disorder is hyperfunctional in nature. Identify this case and the voice disorder involved. Which factors were significant in your choice of disorder?

Exercise 3 Which of the following features is associated with laryngopharyngeal reflux (LPR)?

(a) Cough, dysphonia and throat clearing are infrequent symptoms of LPR.
(b) LPR involves the regurgitation of gastric contents from the proximal oesophagus into the laryngopharynx.
(c) LPR is not believed to play a role in the development of malignant laryngeal carcinoma.
(d) On visual examination, there is inflammation of laryngeal structures indicated by redness and swelling.
(e) LPR can be treated by proton pump inhibitors.

Exercise 4 Which of the following features is *not* associated with muscle tension dysphonia (MTD)?

(a) A glottal gap is frequently observed in clients with MTD.
(b) There is approximation of the false vocal folds in MTD.

(c) Reduced vocal loudness is a common symptom of MTD.

(d) There is increased tension in the (para)laryngeal musculature in MTD.

(e) The larynx can assume an elevated position in the neck of clients with MTD.

Exercise 5 In which of the following scenarios is flexible nasendoscopy used?

(a) The evaluation of velopharyngeal incompetence in the child with cleft palate.

(b) The evaluation of tongue-palate contacts in the child with Down's syndrome.

(c) The evaluation of tongue mobility in the patient with a partial glossectomy.

(d) The evaluation of respiratory function in the adult with Parkinson's disease.

(e) The evaluation of hyponasal voice in an adult with suspected nasal polyps.

7.7 Laryngectomy

Background

A laryngectomy is the surgical removal of the larynx. It is a major, life-altering operation which is usually undertaken to treat laryngeal carcinoma. The larynx can be removed in whole (total laryngectomy) or in part (partial laryngectomy). A lengthy period of recuperation and rehabilitation is necessary in clients who undergo this procedure. Speech and language therapy is a key part of the rehabilitation of these patients. Speech and language therapists will work with patients pre- and post-operatively to establish some alternative means of voice production. Currently, the three main forms of intervention are (a) the use of an electronic or an artificial larynx, (b) the production of oesophageal voice and (c) voice restoration surgery. There is no single best method of intervention, and patients may employ more than one method.

Website

Audiofiles labelled 'Examples of the speaking voices of people who have undergone laryngectomy' can be found at www.cambridge.org/cummings and are used with the permission of the National Association of Laryngectomee Clubs in the UK (www.laryngectomy.org.uk). They contain the speaking voices of six clients who have undergone laryngectomy. These clients are at different stages of their rehabilitation and thus display different levels of proficiency in the use of their chosen method of communication. Listen to the audiofiles several times and then answer the following questions.

Exercise 1 Of the six speakers on the audiofiles, two speakers are using oesophageal voice to communicate, two are using an electronic larynx and two are using a voice prosthesis or a speaking valve. Indicate which method of communication is used by each of these speakers: Don, Bert, Derek, John, Joan, and Stan.

Exercise 2 Three speakers are highly proficient in the use of their chosen method of communication, while three other speakers are less proficient. The latter speakers either have additional complications or are relatively new users of non-laryngeal voice production. List the names of the three speakers with high and low proficiency in the use of their respective methods.

Exercise 3 One of the speakers you have listened to presents with additional complications, as his/her tongue nerve was severed during laryngectomy. Which speaker is this? As a clue to help you identify this speaker, listen to the pronunciation of the word 'communication'.

Exercise 4 Which sound in the production of 'communication' has been compromised by the severed tongue nerve of the client identified in Exercise 3? Why is this sound particularly badly affected?

Exercise 5 Which of the following pairs of adjectives best characterizes Stan's speaking voice: harsh and strangled, wet and gurgly, breathy and quiet?

7.8   Gender dysphoria

Background

In demonstration of the management of transsexual clients, two case studies are presented below. The first case describes a FTM transsexual who received androgen therapy and was followed longitudinally by Van Borsel et al. (2000). The second case describes a MTF transsexual who received hormone and voice therapy and was examined longitudinally by Mount and Salmon (1988).

Case study 1: Subject A (FTM transsexual)

Subject A is a female-to-male transsexual who was aged 22;4 years at the start of the investigation. Before the start of the study, A (a non-smoker) had attempted smoking temporarily in an effort to lower his voice. However, he refrained from further smoking as this had caused him to develop a sore throat. Before hormone therapy commenced, A was consistently mistaken for a female on the telephone. To start with, A received testosterone undecanoate 40 mg twice a day which increased after two months to four times a day. A enjoyed singing and practised for approximately one hour a day.

Data on A were collected on eight occasions for 17 months. When possible, data were collected at intervals of two months – research suggests that virilization of the female voice due to androgynous hormones first becomes evident from 6 to 12 weeks to several months. Two voice therapy sessions took place before androgenic hormones were administered. A's phonational frequency range (lowest and highest pitch level) was determined at each session. A high-quality recording of sustained vowel production (/a/) and A's reading aloud of a standard paragraph was also undertaken. Further acoustic analysis of fundamental frequency, jitter and shimmer was based on this latter recording.

Before androgen therapy commenced, A could phonate at a pitch level >800 Hz. The highest pitch level he could produce after 2.5 months of therapy had decreased to ~660 Hz. His maximum pitch from 4 months post-therapy onwards was in the range 440–525 Hz. Before hormone therapy was initiated, the lowest level he could attain was ~165–175 Hz. This level decreased gradually to ~105 Hz as a result of receiving androgens. During a session 4 months and 10 days after androgen therapy started, it first became apparent that A's fundamental frequency had declined steeply. In the last session, 13 months and 4 days after hormone treatment started, fundamental frequencies of 128 Hz (sustained vowel production) and 155 Hz (reading of paragraph) were recorded.

Male and female voices also differ in vocal jitter and shimmer, with male voices displaying significantly more vocal shimmer and a smaller vocal jitter than the female voice. However, shimmer did not increase or jitter decrease in A as a result of androgen therapy.

Case study 2: Subject B (MTF transsexual)

Subject B is a 63-year-old male-to-female transsexual. B commenced hormone treatment a year before gender reassignment surgery was conducted. She attended a speech clinic for assessment six months after surgery. B reported a low-pitched voice which was not perceived as female, particularly on the telephone. Her speaking voice during conversation and production of sustained vowels was low pitched and appropriate for a bass male speaker. During sustained production of /i, a, u/, B's average fundamental frequency was 110 Hz. B's fundamental frequency at the lowest and highest pitch levels ranged from 110 to 340 Hz.

Voice therapy goals were (a) to train B to use successively higher pitch levels while avoiding vocal abuse and (b) to modify tongue carriage as a means of achieving higher resonance within the vocal tract. The use of a breathy vocal attack and appropriate inflection patterns at higher pitch levels were secondary goals of voice therapy. Words that contained high front vowels and anterior consonants were used in order to increase fundamental frequency and alter resonance characteristics. Words beginning with /h/ were used to establish easy onset of phonation and the use of a breathy voice quality. Phrases and sentences were constructed from these words and used to encourage different types of intonation patterns. To begin with, B listened to the clinician's production and, using Visi-pitch display, attempted to match the pitch contours. In increments of 10 Hz, frequency was raised until B could maintain a consistently good vocal quality at an average fundamental frequency of 210 Hz. Other tasks targeted inflection, resonance and a breathy vocal attack. Role-play situations that emphasized functional conversations were used in the final months of therapy. B was required to engage in conversations in person and over the telephone with people who were unknown to her. In order to assess the appropriateness of vocal behaviours, these conversations were recorded. Telephone work continued until the number of feminine references to B (use of 'Ma'am', for example) predominated.

Treatment extended over 11 months and included 88 one-hour sessions. After four months of therapy, B was able to achieve a fundamental frequency that was comparable to that of females. However, B was not perceived as female on the telephone until six months later. At this time, the altered resonant frequencies of the vocal tract combined with her feminine fundamental frequency were sufficient to elicit female perception. At five years post-treatment, B maintained female vocal characteristics and continued to be perceived as a female on the telephone.

Exercise 1 The fundamental frequency range of men is 98 Hz to 131 Hz, while for women it is 196 Hz to 262 Hz. On the basis of these ranges, how would you characterize the pitch attained by subjects A and B on completion of voice therapy?

Exercise 2 The management of voice in the transsexual patient is as much about avoiding behaviours which may damage the laryngeal apparatus as it is about facilitating new vocal patterns. Do subjects A and B display any behaviours which it is the aim of voice therapy to avert?

Exercise 3 Which of the following statements is an accurate description of vocal jitter and shimmer?

(a) Jitter and shimmer describe the cycle-to-cycle stability of fundamental frequency and amplitude, respectively.
(b) Jitter and shimmer are vocal attributes of adductor spasmodic dysphonia.
(c) Jitter and shimmer are acoustic features of neurogenic voice disorders.
(d) Jitter and shimmer are acoustic features of hyperfunctional voice use.
(e) Jitter and shimmer describe the cycle-to-cycle stability of amplitude and fundamental frequency, respectively.

Exercise 4 The hormone therapy which was received by subject A is described in some detail. Also, subject A's vocal performance is related to different stages in this therapy. This is not the case for subject B. How would you explain this difference?

Exercise 5 How has biofeedback been used within subject B's voice therapy?

SUGGESTIONS FOR FURTHER READING

Adler, R., Hirsch, S. and Mordaunt, M. (eds.) 2012. *Voice and communication therapy for the transgender/transsexual client: a comprehensive clinical guide*, second edition, San Diego, CA: Plural Publishing.

Aronson, A. E. and Bless, D. M. 2009. *Clinical voice disorders*, fourth edition, New York: Thieme (chapters 1, 3, 5 and 8).

Bressmann, T. 2014. 'Head and neck cancer and communication', in L. Cummings (ed.), *Cambridge handbook of communication disorders*, Cambridge: Cambridge University Press, 161–84 (section 10.4 on laryngectomy).

Butcher, P., Elias, A. and Cavalli, L. 2007. *Understanding and treating psychogenic voice disorder: a CBT framework*, Chichester: John Wiley & Sons (chapter 1).

Connor, N. and Bless, N. 2014. 'Functional and organic voice disorders', in L. Cummings (ed.), *Cambridge handbook of communication disorders*, Cambridge: Cambridge University Press, 321–40.

Cummings, L. 2008. *Clinical linguistics*, Edinburgh: Edinburgh University Press (chapter 7).

2014a. *Communication disorders*, Houndmills: Palgrave Macmillan (chapter 7).

Ferrand, C. T. 2012. *Voice disorders: scope of theory and practice*, Pearson (chapters 6 to 12 inclusive).

Haynes, W. O., Moran, M. J. and Pindzola, R. H. 2012. *Communication disorders in educational and medical settings: an introduction for speech-language pathologists, educators and health professionals*, Sudbury, MA: Jones & Bartlett (chapter 9).

Morris, R. and Harmon, A. B. 2013. 'Describing voice disorders', in J. S. Damico, N. Müller and M. J. Ball (eds.), *The handbook of language and speech disorders*, Oxford: Wiley-Blackwell, 455–73.

Chapter 8

Disorders of fluency

Notwithstanding extensive research, stuttering (or stammering) is still one of the least well-understood and successfully remediated communication disorders. Most commonly, the disorder has its onset in the developmental period. There is an increased prevalence of stuttering in association with genetic syndromes. Acquired neurogenic stuttering can occur in adults following a cerebrovascular accident or head trauma (see chapter 6 in Cummings (2008) for further discussion). Cases of acquired psychogenic stuttering have also been reported (see Yaruss (2014) for discussion). In developmental stuttering, the speaker engages in the iteration and protraction of sounds in syllable-initial and word-initial positions. Iterations can involve a single speech sound (e.g. s-s-s-soap) or more than one speech sound, the latter sound typically a schwa vowel (e.g. sə-sə-sə-side). Protractions or perseverations are always single speech sounds (e.g. s::::soap). Alongside these speech features, the person who stutters may also display secondary or accessory behaviours. These behaviours may be verbal or non-verbal in nature and include eye blinking, avoidance of eye contact, silent rehearsal and substitution of one word for another (e.g. officer of the law for 'policeman'). The person who stutters may not be aware of these secondary behaviours. Certainly, they are addressed alongside speech features in the assessment and treatment of stuttering.

Cluttering is a less well-known fluency disorder than stuttering. It may occur alongside stuttering in the same person and is often confused for stuttering by professionals and lay people alike. The disorder has been reported in several syndromes (e.g. fragile X syndrome) and has also been linked to brain damage in adults (Cummings, 2008). The chief speech feature of cluttering is a rapid and/or irregular rate of speech. Other features include excessive non-stuttering-like dysfluencies, excessive collapsing or deletion of syllables, and abnormal pauses, syllable stress, or speech rhythm (Scaler Scott, 2014). It has been widely remarked that the person who clutters is unaware of their difficulties with fluency. However, the reports of people with cluttering suggest that this may not be the case (Scaler Scott, 2014). Notwithstanding the widespread neglect of this fluency disorder, even to the point of the denial of its existence, there is now a sustained research effort underway to obtain an accurate definition of cluttering with a view to performing a differential diagnosis of the disorder (Scaler Scott, 2014).

Section A: Short-answer questions

8.1 Developmental stuttering

(1) Fill in the blank spaces in these paragraphs using the words in the box below:
Although much has been written about stuttering in children, remarkably little progress has been made to date in understanding the causes of this disorder. Explanations of the cause of this disorder include _____, psychological and environmental factors. What is clear is that more males than females experience this communication disorder – the ratio of stuttering males to females is around _____ in very young

preschool children and _____ in adults. It is also known that children who have first-degree relatives who stutter are _____ times more likely to go on to develop a stutter. Although figures vary, it is also the case that for a large number of children who develop stuttering, the problem can _____ spontaneously.

The speech features of stuttering have been extensively described. We know, for example, that the _____ and _____ that occur in stuttering are qualitatively distinct from the nonfluencies that occur in normal speech. The child who stutters repeats speech elements of less than a full _____. Such an element may be a single _____ as in /ʃ/ of 'ship' or a phoneme and _____ combination as in /ka/ for 'cap'. These speech elements may also be prolonged beyond their normal _____, e.g. /ʃːː/ for 'ship' and /kaːːː/ for 'cap'. Other speech behaviours of the stutterer include the insertion of a word such as 'really', known as a _____, in advance of a word that may cause the stutterer to block. The stutterer may also insert a _____ before a sound or word that is likely to be problematic.

Stutterers are also adept at talking around words that are likely to cause them difficulty (e.g. use of 'officer of the law' for *policeman*). This behaviour is known as _____. This avoidance of words may be part of a wider avoidance of people and speaking situations in the person who is a _____ stutterer. A person with _____ or covert stuttering may appear fluent to listeners. Several non-verbal behaviours, variously called _____ or accessory features, can attend stuttering behaviour. These behaviours include sudden loss of eye contact, rapid eye blinking, hand tapping, head nodding, jaw jerk, tongue thrust and nostril flaring. In some cases, these behaviours can be extreme and are more evident to the listener than the _____ itself.

interiorized	syllable	neologism	phoneme		
consonant	iterations	schwa	pet starter		
five	three	2:1	10:1	4:1	7:1
overt	chromosomal		resolve	perseverations	
genetic	secondaries	vowel	circumlocution	duration	
dysfluency	covert	normal non-fluency		avoidance	

(2) Which of the following is *not* a true statement about the epidemiology of developmental stuttering?
(a) Developmental stuttering has a general population prevalence of 5%.
(b) Prevalence figures decrease with increasing age.
(c) The male-to-female sex ratio is approximately 4:1.
(d) Prevalence rates are higher in certain special populations (e.g. children and adults with Down's syndrome) than in the general population.
(e) The prevalence of developmental stuttering is consistent across countries and cultures.

(3) Which of the following is *not* a true statement about the aetiology of developmental stuttering?
(a) The aetiology of developmental stuttering is still unknown.
(b) There is now a general consensus that parenting styles do not play a causal role in the development of stuttering.

(c) A genetic basis for the disorder is supported by studies which have found an increased rate of stuttering in the biological relatives of stutterers.

(d) A neurological basis for the disorder is supported by MRI studies which have identified lesions in the region of Broca's area.

(e) The aetiology of developmental stuttering is likely to be multifactorial in nature.

(4) *True* or *False*: Approximately 75% of children who stutter recover spontaneously from the disorder.

(5) *True* or *False*: The child who stutters often exhibits developmental problems in other domains (e.g. socialization).

(6) Which of the following is a speech feature of developmental stuttering?
   (a) Speech exhibits iterations of word-initial phonemes.
   (b) Speech exhibits protractions of word-final phonemes.
   (c) Iterations can involve a schwa vowel.
   (d) Iterations and protractions are always audible.
   (e) Speech displays an excessive rate.

(7) Which of the following is a *true* statement about accessory features in developmental stuttering?
   (a) Accessory features include verbal and non-verbal behaviours.
   (b) Facial grimacing and eye blinking are common accessory features.
   (c) The function of accessory features is to distract the listener from the speaker's stuttering behaviour.
   (d) The relationship of accessory features to stuttering behaviour is uncertain.
   (e) The person who stutters is always aware of the accessory features that attend their stuttering.

(8) *True* or *False*: Three-quarters of people who stutter started doing so before the age of 6 years.

(9) Which of the following areas are of interest to a speech and language therapist who is assessing a child referred to SLT services because of a concern about stuttering?
   (a) The therapist needs to establish if language skills are age-appropriate.
   (b) During the taking of a personal history, the therapist will want to establish if biological relatives of the child stutter.
   (c) The therapist will want to assess the phonetic inventory of the child and establish that phonological skills are age-appropriate.
   (d) The therapist will assess the child's gross motor skills.
   (e) The therapist will assess the child's feeding skills and ability to swallow.

(10) Which of the following statements characterize treatment of the child who stutters?
   (a) Group therapy has limited effectiveness in the treatment of stuttering in children.
   (b) Fluency can be established relatively quickly in treatment programmes but there is frequent relapse once therapy has ended.
   (c) Therapy aims to encourage children to reflect on their feelings and attitudes towards stuttering.
   (d) There is an emphasis on improving the speed, range and accuracy of articulatory movements for speech during treatment.
   (e) Children can be taught how to use a number of speech modification techniques (e.g. soft glottal onsets).

8.2   Acquired stuttering

(1) *True* or *False*: The adult who stutters may have either persistent developmental stuttering or acquired stuttering.

(2) *True* or *False*: Acquired stuttering can be neurogenic or psychogenic in nature.

(3) *True* or *False*: Acquired stuttering is more prevalent than developmental stuttering.

(4) Which of the following is *not* a cause of acquired stuttering?
   (a) traumatic brain injury
   (b) cerebrovascular accident
   (c) Alzheimer's disease
   (d) progressive supranuclear palsy
   (e) subcortical damage

(5) Some researchers believe it is possible to identify features which distinguish neurogenic stuttering from developmental stuttering in adults. Which of the following features do researchers believe can be used for this purpose?
   (a) Only in neurogenic stuttering is the speaker frustrated and anxious.
   (b) Only in neurogenic stuttering do repetitions, prolongations and blocks not occur solely on initial syllables of words and utterances.
   (c) Only in developmental stuttering are secondary symptoms not associated with moments of dysfluency.
   (d) Only in developmental stuttering do dysfluencies occur on grammatical words nearly as frequently as on substantive words.
   (e) Only in developmental stuttering is the speaker aware of dysfluencies.

(6) Fill in the blank spaces in this paragraph using the words in the box below:
The communication problems which result from acquired brain damage are most often a motor speech disorder such as _____ or a language disorder like aphasia. Less commonly, the onset of stuttering occurs in an adult who sustains a _____, a traumatic brain injury or other _____ event. It is often difficult to distinguish the dysfluency of acquired stuttering from the dysfluencies associated with dysarthria and _____. It is also difficult to identify the brain _____ site that gives rise to acquired stuttering. In fact, with the exception of the occipital lobe, most cortical and _____ areas have been implicated in neurogenic stuttering. A further challenge to the characterization of acquired stuttering is that in some cases there is a _____ rather than a neuropathological origin of the disorder.

lesion	aphasia	brainstem	subcortical
infarction	seizure	psychological	dysarthria
haemorrhage	stroke	cognitive	neurological

(7) Which of the following are *true* statements about acquired stuttering?
   (a) Acquired stuttering is less successfully treated than developmental stuttering.
   (b) A prior communication disorder is a risk factor for acquired stuttering.
   (c) Acquired neurogenic stuttering has been associated with brain dysfunction secondary to anorexia nervosa.
   (d) Acquired stuttering always occurs in the presence of a language disorder.
   (e) Acquired stuttering may have a neuropsychiatric origin.

(8) *True* or *False*: Singing and chorus speaking can induce immediate fluency in developmental, but not neurogenic, stuttering.

(9) *True* or *False*: There is evidence that professionals in fluency disorders can fail to reliably distinguish speakers with developmental stuttering from speakers with neurogenic stuttering on the basis of speech features alone.

(10) *True* or *False*: Acquired neurogenic stuttering always occurs in the presence of apraxia of speech.

8.3   Cluttering

(1) Which of the following statements characterize the fluency disorder of cluttering?
  (a) Cluttering is a more prevalent disorder than stuttering, particularly in children.
  (b) The person who clutters displays little awareness of his or her fluency problems.
  (c) Cluttering and stuttering may co-exist in the same individual.
  (d) Speaking rate is markedly deviant in cluttering.
  (e) Cluttering is frequently misdiagnosed as stuttering.

(2) *True* or *False*: There is evidence of language problems in cluttering.

(3) *True* or *False*: Cluttering has been reported to occur in several syndromes including Tourette's syndrome and fragile X syndrome.

(4) *True* or *False*: Cluttering is not associated with acquired brain damage in adults.

(5) Which of the following features should alert clinicians to the need to evaluate a client further for cluttering?
  (a) the presence of disorganized language
  (b) the presence of an auditory comprehension deficit
  (c) rapid or fluctuating speech rate
  (d) the presence of neologisms in spoken output
  (e) the presence of verbal perseveration in spoken output

(6) Investigators have attempted to establish features which can be used in a differential diagnosis of cluttering. Which of the following features have been discussed with a view to distinguishing cluttering from stuttering?
  (a) People who clutter have lower mean pause times than people who stutter.
  (b) People who clutter have greater mean phonation times than people who stutter.
  (c) Multiple repetitions of words and phrases are never found in people who clutter, only in people who stutter.
  (d) Writing problems and poor handwriting are never found in people who clutter, only in people who stutter.
  (e) People who clutter have no awareness of their problems with communication.

(7) *True* or *False*: Cluttering is still not recognized as a diagnostic category in the *Diagnostic and Statistical Manual of Mental Disorders* or by the World Health Organization.

(8) *True* or *False*: The person who clutters may exhibit excessive non-stuttering-like disfluencies.

(9) Efforts are continuing to arrive at a satisfactory definition of cluttering. The three features which most clinicians appear to agree are core cluttering symptoms include anomalies of _____, fluency and speech clarity.

(10) There has been little systematic investigation of the _____ of cluttering. However, on the basis of those studies which have been conducted, the disorder is known to be more common in males than in females.

Section B: Data analysis exercises

8.4 Developmental stuttering

Background

NS is a 24-year-old male who has been stuttering since childhood (Ball et al., 2009). He displays excessive struggle behaviours and facial grimacing during spontaneous speech. The following data are taken from a recording of NS reading a passage about the football World Cup in Spain. In order to illustrate the strategies that NS uses to get beyond his repetitions, the transcription uses symbols from the Extended International Phonetic Alphabet (extIPA) and the Voice Quality Symbols system (VoQS).

Data

'the World Cup': [ð\ð:ə̣ {V̰ ə\ə\ə V̰} 'hw̰əɹld 'kʌp]
'the top nations': [ðə tˢ \tᵈ (.) {p t'\t' p} fŋ\ {ʃfŋ\fŋʃ} \'t̪ɒ̈p' 'neʃənz]
'in a tournament': [ɪn·ə̣ {pp tʰ·əʃ\t̃ʰə\təʃpp}\'t̪ʉɹnəmənt]
'provincial towns': [p\pɹəv\'vɪnʃəl {p t'\t' p} \ {pp t'\t' pp} (.) t'\t' {pp t'\t' pp} fŋ\fŋ \ {↓'tã̈ʊ̃nz ↓}]
'the semi-finals': [ðə s'\s'\s'\'s' {↓ɛmi 'faɪnəlz↓}]

Exercise 1 As is typically the case in stuttering, NS displays marked dysfluency in the form of repetitions of word-initial sounds. Which two classes of sounds are most affected during these repetitions?

Exercise 2 Repetitions in NS's speech are characterized by anomalies of voice quality. Where in the data do these anomalies occur?

Exercise 3 Articulations involving non-English sounds are sometimes evident during repetitions in NS's speech. An example of such a sound occurs during the production of 'the top nations' and 'provincial towns'. In what other clinical population is this sound often found?

Exercise 4 Prosodic disturbances involving loudness are evident in NS's repetitions. Using the data provided, characterize these disturbances.

Exercise 5 Airstream anomalies are also evident in NS's speech. These anomalies include the use of non-pulmonic sounds known as ejectives as well as pulmonic ingressive sounds. Give <u>two</u> examples of each type of production in the data. What do they indicate about NS's use of breath support for speech?

8.5   Acquired stuttering 1

Background

Mower and Younts (2001) describe a case of neurogenic stuttering in the presence of a neurodegenerative disease, namely, multiple sclerosis (MS). The patient, a 36-year-old man known as SS, was hospitalized for the treatment of MS. In August 1994, SS displayed sudden onset of excessive word repetitions. An MRI scan performed in September 1994 was consistent with his MS condition (i.e. plaques were seen in the white matter involving the medulla, cerebellum, basal ganglion and periventricular white matter). A small, irregular corpus callosum was also noted. Some of SS's dysfluent speech is presented below in orthographic and phonetic transcription.

Well, we-we-we-we-we in-in-in port mo-most of time and-and when-when-when I got-got married, got-got-got-got-got-got an apar-par-partment.

Target	Client production
load	[lo.lo.lod]
crates	[krei.krei.krei.kreits]
with	[wə.wə.wɪə]
most	[mo.most.most]
Monday	[mə.mə.mən.dei]
navy	[nei.nei.nei.vi]
supplies	[sə.sə.sə.plaiz]
side	[sai.said]

Exercise 1 Two forms of repetition are particularly common in SS's speech. What are these forms? How would you characterize the linguistic units involved in these repetitions, and do they differ from the units which undergo repetition in developmental stuttering?

Exercise 2 Are sound prolongations or perseverations a feature of SS's speech? In what form of stuttering are these sound errors found?

Exercise 3 In developmental stuttering, part-word repetition leads into the fluent production of multisyllabic target words in their entirety. Does this occur in SS's case? Use data to support your answer.

Exercise 4 The word 'apartment' is one of several unusual repetition sequences produced by SS. In what way is it unusual?

Exercise 5 Other examples of the unusual repetition sequence identified in Example 4 were 'hopefully' (hope-hopeful-fully), 'supervisors' (su-su-su-supervi-vi-visors), 'overboard' (overbo-bo-board), 'Mediterranean' (Me-me-medit-ter-ter-ter-anean), 'appointment' (a-puh-puh-pointment) and 'parachute' (par-par-parachute-chute). One of these repetitions differs slightly from the others. Which repetition is it and in what way is it different?

8.5 Acquired stuttering 2

Clinicians must consider a range of organic and other factors in the differential diagnosis of acquired neurogenic and psychogenic stuttering in adults. The following case study describes a 29-year-old white male, who began stuttering secondary to psychological stress. Examine the details of this case and then answer the questions below.

Case study

Background

A, a graphic designer at a university, was referred by his primary care physician to speech pathology following an acute onset of dysfluent speech. There was no prior history of stuttering. With the exception of his father, who had had complex partial seizures since his early 20s (he was now 58 years old), there was also no family history of neurological disease.

Presenting symptoms

A reported that his first episode of stuttering occurred on the word 'paper', an item integral to his work. Throughout the morning of the following day his dysfluencies increased, and by early afternoon of that day he was severely dysfluent. The pitch of his voice also increased during a period of three to four days, before returning to normal over the next month. A was unable to write in capital letters, although lower-case letters and cursive writing were intact. After seven days, A's problem with writing resolved spontaneously. A reported that he had been under stress for the last few months. His presenting symptoms appeared to be consistent with a diagnosis of conversion reaction. Neurological evaluations undertaken at this time, which included EEG, MRI, CT scans and lumbar puncture, were all normal.

Speech evaluation

A underwent a speech evaluation 19 days after the onset of stuttering. His speech was judged to be severely dysfluent. He displayed frequent syllable and word repetitions, with infrequent blocks on syllables and words. During conversational speech and oral reading, every syllable and word exhibited multiple repetitions. As many as 20 or more repetitions per syllable were routinely noted. The stuttering pattern did not alter during choral reading. Even when mouthing words without voicing during conversational speech and reading, stuttering was exhibited. A displayed increased pitch which was secondary to tension observed in the shoulder and neck areas. There were no starters or secondary characteristics, no specific word fears or avoidances and no situational fears (e.g. use of the telephone). There were no changes reported in cognitive function and expressive and receptive language. No limb tremors or lingual fasciculations were observed at this time. Fluency therapy was commenced three times a week and lasted for three months. Although A demonstrated self-control of stuttered and fluent speech production, and his pitch returned to normal, his dysfluent speech subsequently became more severe, and other motor anomalies (e.g. lingual fasciculations and hand and leg tremors) appeared for the first time. A second referral to neurology was made.

Neurology

Normal proportions of dopamine were shown on single-photon emission computed tomography (SPECT) scanning. There was a normal cranial nerve examination apart from markedly slow tongue movements. A sensory examination to all primary and cortical modalities was normal. During a cerebellar examination, there were normal finger to nose movements in procession, although movements were slow. A tremor persisted during these movements but did not increase in amplitude. A motor examination revealed a tremor at rest in both arms (right more than left), and a slight tremor in the right leg at rest. A was able to stand, but he could not walk on his heels and toes. Balance was judged to be slightly abnormal, and his face was without expression. Movements were slow to begin and to complete. He was unable to execute rapid, alternating movements.

Most of A's clinical features were suggestive of parkinsonism. Carbidopa-levodopa was prescribed with dose reductions made as improvements occurred in speech and motor skills. However, when the dose was reduced to a certain level, A's stuttering was observed to increase in severity.

Psychiatry

Based upon the initial diagnosis of a conversion reaction, psychiatric intervention was commenced. A psychiatrist prescribed medication for depression and sleep. Behavioural and psychiatric strategies to improve A's stuttering were discussed by the psychiatrist and speech-language pathologist during twice weekly telephone calls. However, psychiatric intervention resulted in no improvement in A's stuttering and the psychiatrist believed the disorder to be organic in nature.

Exercise 1 List five ways in which A's stuttering behaviour differs from that seen in developmental stuttering.

Exercise 2 Which of the following clinical features of parkinsonism might account for A's problems with writing?

(a) festination
(b) micrographia
(c) rest tremor
(d) bradykinesia
(e) rigidity

Exercise 3 Psychogenic stuttering caused by a conversion reaction was an early diagnosis of A's disorder. What features of this case make this a plausible, albeit mistaken, diagnosis of A's condition?

Exercise 4 A's face was without expression and is consistent with parkinsonian facies. Which of the following statements characterizes this clinical feature of parkinsonism?

(a) The lack of facial expressiveness is caused by the rigidity of facial muscles.
(b) The lack of facial expressiveness is a sign of emotional lability.
(c) The lack of facial expressiveness has an adverse impact on a client's communication skills.

(d) The lack of facial expressiveness is related to auditory comprehension problems.
(e) The lack of facial expressiveness is related to cognitive deficits.

Exercise 5 During his neurological examination, A displays dysdiadochokinesia. Which of the following behaviours does this term describe?

(a) the slow initiation of movement
(b) a rest tremor in both arms
(c) slow tongue movements
(d) an inability to walk on one's heels and toes
(e) an inability to carry out rapid alternating movements

8.6   Cluttering

Background

Reflecting the fact that cluttering has both motoric and linguistic components, Ward (2006: 144) distinguishes between motoric and linguistic cluttering. Examples of the speech produced in each type of cluttering are shown below. The speaker in (A) is an 18-year-old male. His verbal output is characterized by fast rushes of speech (the symbol (:) represents short pauses). The speaker in (B) is a 25-year-old male. His speech rate is mostly within normal limits.

Speaker A: *Motoric cluttering*

Normally I c c come by car, but t t t today I (:) took the bus. My car (:) had to go for a (:) service.

Speaker B: *Linguistic cluttering*

My, favourite – well, the best, best place for my, for a holiday is um, um, is, er, Australia. The heat, well, the er, the er, climate really is . . . . It's it's really great.

Exercise 1 On the basis of the above data, describe two features of motoric cluttering which are not related to speech rate.

Exercise 2 On the basis of the above data, describe two features of linguistic cluttering which are not related to speech rate.

Exercise 3 Are any of the features you have identified in response to Exercises 1 and 2 also a feature of stuttering?

Exercise 4 The verbal output of speaker B is not unlike that found in some other clinical conditions (e.g. aphasia). What specific linguistic difficulty is suggested by this output?

Exercise 5 The pauses used by speaker A are unlike those found in normal speech. Explain the feature which distinguishes speaker A's pauses from those produced by speakers who do not clutter.

SUGGESTIONS FOR FURTHER READING

Cummings, L. 2008. *Clinical linguistics*, Edinburgh: Edinburgh University Press (chapter 6).
2014a. *Communication disorders*, Houndmills: Palgrave Macmillan (chapter 8).

Haynes, W. O., Moran, M. J. and Pindzola, R. H. 2012. *Communication disorders in educational and medical settings: an introduction for speech-language pathologists, educators and health professionals*, Sudbury, MA: Jones & Bartlett (chapter 8).

Lundgren, K., Helm-Estabrooks, N. and Klein, R. 2010. 'Stuttering following acquired brain damage: a review of the literature', *Journal of Neurolinguistics* **23**:5, 447–54.

Scaler Scott, K. 2014. 'Stuttering and cluttering', in L. Cummings (ed.), *Cambridge handbook of communication disorders*, Cambridge: Cambridge University Press, 341–58.

Silverman, F. H. 2004. *Stuttering and other fluency disorders*, Long Grove, IL: Waveland Press, Inc.

Tetnowski, J. A. and Scaler Scott, K. 2013. 'Fluency and fluency disorders', in J. S. Damico, N. Müller and M. J. Ball (eds.), *The handbook of language and speech disorders*, Oxford: Wiley-Blackwell, 431–54.

Van Borsel, J. and Tetnowski, J. A. 2007. 'Fluency disorders in genetic syndromes', *Journal of Fluency Disorders* **32**:4, 279–96.

Ward, D. 2006. *Stuttering and cluttering: frameworks for understanding and treatment*, Hove: Psychology Press (chapters 1, 8 and 16).

Ward, D. and Scaler Scott, K. (eds.) 2011. *Cluttering: a handbook of research, intervention and education*, Hove: Psychology Press (parts 1 and 2).

Chapter 9

Hearing disorders

Hearing disorders can result from damage to the ear, the auditory pathways to the brain and the auditory cortices of the brain. Depending on the location of this damage, a child or adult may be said to have a conductive or sensorineural hearing loss. If there is damage to the outer or middle ear, a conductive hearing loss is often the result. For example, the ear canal or external auditory meatus may fail to develop normally during embryological development in conditions such as Treacher Collins syndrome. A severe conductive hearing loss occurs when there is complete atresia of the ear canal. Alternatively, the palatal abnormalities of the child with a cleft palate may compromise the opening of the Eustachian tube, leading to reduced ventilation of the middle ear. (The contraction of the tensor veli palatini muscle causes this tube to open.) This can lead to the development of otitis media ('glue ear') in which a conductive hearing loss arises from impaired mechanical vibration of the ossicular chain in the middle ear. This disorder can be treated by means of the insertion of a pressure equalizing tube into the tympanic membrane in a surgical procedure known as a myringotomy. In another middle ear disorder known as otosclerosis, new bone growth on the anterior footplate of the stapes (the third bone in the ossicular chain) can cause a conductive hearing loss of up to 50 dB (Ackley, 2014).

Even when the conduction of sound waves through the external and middle ear is successfully achieved, a range of inner ear problems can impede normal hearing. For example, hair cells in the cochlea may be damaged as a result of infections such as meningitis. Also, the stereocilia of these cells may become fractured following sustained noise exposure. In both cases, the generation of nervous impulses from the inner ear along the auditory pathway to the brain will be compromised. Parts of this pathway may also be damaged as a result of infections, trauma or cerebrovascular accidents. The auditory cortices which receive nervous signals from the inner ear may be impaired following a head trauma or cerebrovascular accident. In each of these scenarios, the child or adult will experience a sensorineural hearing loss which may be partial or complete. Where a sensorineural hearing loss is related to cochlear damage, treatment may involve cochlea implantation. In the assessment and treatment of hearing disorders, speech and language therapists must work closely with audiologists and ENT specialists (otolaryngologists) as part of a multidisciplinary team.

Section A: Short-answer questions

9.1 Conductive hearing loss

(1) For each statement below, indicate if a conductive or sensorineural hearing loss is described:
  (a) A child with cleft palate has impaired hearing after recurrent episodes of otitis media.
  (b) A 2-year-old child, who sustains a head injury, experiences hearing loss.
  (c) An adult develops hearing loss following severe meningococcal infection.

(d) A 45-year-old man is diagnosed as having a hearing loss related to otosclerosis.

(e) A child with Apert's syndrome has bilateral hearing loss on audiological assessment.

(2) Fill in the blank spaces in this paragraph using words in the box below:

Otitis media is a common _____ infection in children. The disorder arises when the _____ fails to ventilate the middle ear adequately. This scenario is frequently encountered in children with a _____, where defects of palatal muscles such as the _____ limit the opening of the Eustachian tube. In the absence of sufficient _____, fluid can build up in the middle ear. This fluid dampens the mechanical vibration of the three _____ in the middle ear. The bones which make up the ossicular chain are called the _____, incus and _____. They are noteworthy on account of being the _____ bones in the human body. Sometimes the fluid in the middle ear becomes infected with bacteria, leading to the development of _____ otitis media. The only route of escape for this infected fluid in the middle ear is to burst through the _____ and exit along the _____ or ear canal. To avoid repeated _____ of the ear drum in children with cleft palate, the otolaryngologist will perform a surgical procedure known as a _____. This is where a small incision is made in the tympanic membrane into which is inserted a ventilating tube or a _____ tube. This tube assumes the role of ventilating the _____ and is naturally expelled by the ear after a period of some months.

external auditory meatus	stapes	outer ear	smallest
ventilation	perforations	Eustachian tube	stapedectomy
cleft palate	tympanometry	incus	suppurative
tympanic membrane	round window		tensor veli palatini
pressure-equalizing	middle ear	pinna	malleus
oval window	ossicles	myringotomy	stapedius muscle

(3) Which of the following is *true* of complete ear canal atresia?
   (a) It appears on a CAT scan as no airway to the tympanic membrane.
   (b) It is often found in individuals with Treacher Collins syndrome.
   (c) It involves stenosis of the ear canal.
   (d) It is associated with sensorineural hearing loss.
   (e) It often indicates the presence of middle ear pathology.

(4) Which of the following statements about cholesteatoma is *false*?
   (a) Cholesteatoma erodes the ossicles in the middle ear.
   (b) Cholesteatoma is a malignant accumulation of epithelium in the middle ear.
   (c) Cholesteatoma can be a complication of the perforation of the tympanic membrane.
   (d) Treatment involves surgical removal of the cholesteatoma and ossicular reconstruction.
   (e) Cholesteatoma grows superiorly in the attic of the tympanic membrane.

(5) Which of the following statements is *true* of otosclerosis?
   (a) Otosclerosis is an inner ear disorder.
   (b) Otosclerosis causes sensorineural hearing loss.
   (c) Otosclerosis is caused by new bone growth on the malleus.

    (d) Stapedectomy is the treatment of choice for otosclerosis.

    (e) Otosclerosis impedes the movement of the stapes.

(6) Middle ear pressure and Eustachian tube function can be assessed by means of: pure tone audiometry, tympanometry, auditory brainstem response testing (underline one).

(7) When bone conduction hearing is better than air conduction hearing during pure tone audiometry, the audiologist will diagnose: conductive hearing loss, sensorineural hearing loss, central auditory processing disorder (underline one).

(8) Respond with *true* or *false* to each of the following statements:

    (a) Hearing loss which is related to a craniofacial defect is most often sensorineural in nature.

    (b) The tensor veli palatini and levator veli palatini muscles act on the Eustachian tube to achieve ventilation of the middle ear.

    (c) Glomus jugulare tumour is a malignant growth in the middle ear.

    (d) Hearing loss which is related to ossification of the stapes is conductive in nature.

    (e) Middle ear squamous cell carcinoma is the most common malignancy of the ear.

(9) Which of the following is a significant cause of conductive hearing loss in children?

    (a) maternal rubella

    (b) meningitis

    (c) malformations of the pinna

    (d) stenotic ear canal

    (e) recurrent otitis media

(10) In which of the following syndromes is conductive hearing loss a clinical feature?

    (a) foetal alcohol syndrome

    (b) Landau-Kleffner syndrome

    (c) Treacher Collins syndrome

    (d) Wolf-Hirschhorn syndrome

    (e) Asperger's syndrome

9.2   Sensorineural hearing loss

(1) Which of the following is a cause of sensorineural hearing loss?

    (a) meningitis

    (b) otitis media

    (c) maternal rubella

    (d) auditory canal atresia

    (e) some antibiotics

(2) Presbycusis is a common cause of sensorineural hearing loss in adulthood. Which of the following statements are *true* of this disorder?

    (a) Presbycusis is an age-related deterioration of the cochlea and auditory nerve.

    (b) Presbycusis seldom involves high frequency hearing.

    (c) Recruitment is a rare symptom of presbycusis.

    (d) In cochlear conductive presbycusis, the elasticity and flexibility of cochlear tissue are compromised.

    (e) Basal hair cells are lost in presbycusis.

(3) Fill in the blank spaces in this paragraph using words in the box below:

Noise exposure is a leading cause of _____ in adults, particularly in industrialized societies. Hearing is _____ in the 125–8000 Hz frequency range with the exception of the 4000 Hz frequency. One symptom of the disorder, which can impair sleep and mental health, is _____. Other symptoms include poor speech understanding, recruitment (an _____ to loud sound) and impaired _____ hearing. The _____ base is the first region of the ear to be damaged. The hair cells, which are responsible for 4000 Hz signals, are located 8–10 mm from the base of the _____ membrane. When noise is not tolerated, the _____ of these cells fracture. As noise exposure continues, the stereocilia are expelled and atrophy of the _____ occurs. This damage is irreversible and affected individuals experience a permanent _____ in hearing. Noise exposure may be the reason that _____ develops.

semicircular	cell body	normal	presbycusis
hearing loss	otosclerosis	threshold shift	
vestibular	intolerance	stereocilia	tinnitus
recruitment	cochlear	directional	basilar

(4) Which of the following statements are *true* claims about the ototoxic effects of drugs?
  (a) Aminoglycoside antibiotics can cause permanent hearing loss.
  (b) Streptomycin, an antibiotic which is used to treat tuberculosis, is more frequently vestibulotoxic than ototoxic.
  (c) The destruction of cochlear hair cells is not among the ototoxic effects of neomycin.
  (d) Certain diuretics can produce irreversible auditory symptoms.
  (e) Aspirin does not have ototoxic effects.

(5) Which of the following statements are *true* claims about Ménière's disease?
  (a) Ménière's disease is a middle ear disorder.
  (b) Hearing loss is sensorineural in nature and fluctuates in the low frequencies.
  (c) Aural pressure is not a symptom of the disease.
  (d) Tinnitus and vertigo are symptoms of Ménière's disease.
  (e) Excessive production of endolymph is believed to be the pathophysiological mechanism of the disease.

(6) An acoustic reflex test is sensitive to the presence of: cholesteatoma, acoustic nerve tumour, otosclerosis (underline one).

(7) The middle latency response gives electrophysiological data corresponding to the activity of the: vestibular cochlear nerve, auditory cortical centres, tympanic membrane (underline one).

(8) Through the measurement of otoacoustic emissions audiologists can diagnose: conductive hearing loss, sensorineural hearing loss, reduced eardrum mobility (underline one).

(9) Prenatal exposure to alcohol can have significant ototoxic effects. This can be seen in children with foetal alcohol syndrome, where a range of hearing problems can occur as a result of exposure to alcohol. Identify these problems among the list below:
  (a) central auditory processing disorder
  (b) ossification of the stapes

      (c) conductive hearing loss

      (d) perforation of the tympanic membrane

      (e) sensorineural hearing loss

(10) Respond with *True* or *False* to each of the following statements:

      (a) A vestibular schwannoma is a malignant tumour of the vestibular cochlear nerve.

      (b) Tinnitus is a rare auditory symptom which is typically only found in noise-induced hearing loss.

      (c) Auditory processing disorder has a high prevalence in children with learning disability and reading disorder.

      (d) Hearing loss which is related to damage of cochlear hair cells is conductive in nature.

      (e) Sound localization and auditory discrimination are both types of central auditory processing.

9.3   Cochlear implantation

(1) *True* or *False*: The cochlear implant is a surgically inserted device that delivers electrical stimulation to the inner ear and fifth cranial nerve.

(2) Which of the following children with hearing loss benefit from a cochlear implant?

      (a) The child who has damaged cochlear hair cells and an intact auditory nerve following meningococcal infection.

      (b) The child with sensorineural hearing loss related to an acoustic neuroma.

      (c) The child with Treacher Collins syndrome who has complete atresia of the ear canal.

      (d) The child with cleft palate who experiences recurrent episodes of otitis media.

      (e) The child with cochlear aplasia who has an absent cochlea.

(3) Which of the following statements is *true* of speech and language outcomes following cochlear implantation in children?

      (a) Children who undergo implantation at younger ages are more accurate on average in their production of consonants, vowels, intonation and rhythm than children who undergo the procedure at older ages.

      (b) At one year after implantation, speech intelligibility is twice that reported for children with profound hearing impairments.

      (c) Speech produced by children who receive implants is more accurate than speech produced by children who have comparable hearing losses and use other devices.

      (d) Improvements in speech intelligibility decline markedly one year after implantation.

      (e) Oral language development does not display the improvements seen in speech intelligibility.

(4) *True* or *False*: Cochlear implantation is not suitable for children who lose their hearing before developing speech and language.

(5) *True* or *False*: Cochlear implants are successfully used in the management of meningitic paediatric patients.

(6) Which of the following statements is *true* of adults with cochlear implants?

      (a) Prelingually deafened adults demonstrate poorer speech perception skills with an implant than postlingually deafened adults.

(b) Prelingually deafened adults demonstrate little change in postoperative speech recognition over time.

(c) Prelingually deafened adults demonstrate significant improvements in postoperative speech production over time, even in the absence of intensive rehabilitation.

(d) Prelingually deafened adults demonstrate a higher rate of device non-use than postlingually deafened adults.

(e) Most postlingually deafened adults demonstrate significantly enhanced lip-reading skills when using a cochlear implant.

(7) Fill in the blank spaces in these paragraphs using the words in the box below:

Several factors are known to affect the performance of children with cochlear implants. These factors include age at onset of profound deafness, status of the _____, age when the child receives the implant, the presence of additional _____, the amount of residual hearing prior to implantation and the child's _____ environment. Postlingually deafened children demonstrate _____ gains with cochlear implants than prelingually deafened children. This difference is due to the greater experience with sound in _____ deafened children. _____ malformations of the cochlea may affect the performance of children with a cochlear implant but do not exclude these children as candidates for the procedure.

Children who receive an implant at an early age tend to outperform children who receive an implant later. Earlier implantation maximizes the amount of auditory information which is available to the child during the _____ for language learning. Additional disabilities such as _____ disability secondary to _____ can affect children's performance with a cochlear implant. There is also evidence that the type of educational environment can affect the performance of children with implants. Although there is disagreement on the type of environment which achieves the best performance – for example, _____ communication programs or _____ communication settings – most professionals agree that schools should provide an optimal auditory environment for children in order to promote _____ development.

prelingually	quicker	congenital	disabilities	
critical period	phonological	educational	total	
reading	postlingually	verbal	auditory	meningitis
intellectual	non-verbal	cochlea	oral	genetic

(8) *True* or *False*: For a child to be a candidate to receive a cochlear implant, he or she must have severe-to-profound bilateral sensorineural hearing loss.

(9) Which of the following factors make the child with Down's syndrome an unsuitable candidate to receive a cochlear implant?

(a) recurrent episodes of otitis media

(b) an intellectual disability

(c) intolerance of the device

(d) conductive hearing loss

(e) craniofacial anomalies

(10) A contraindication for cochlear implants in children is deafness due to lesions of the _____ auditory pathway.

Section B: Data analysis exercises

9.4   Congenital hearing loss 1

Background

The following data are taken from recordings and transcriptions of 10 sentences read by 40 deaf children aged between 8 and 15 years (Smith, 1975). These children were all of normal intelligence and had no apparent anomalies other than deafness. A range of interjected sounds characterize these children's productions.

Target word(s)	Client production	Target word(s)	Client production
mean to	[min ə stu]	swim	[dəwɪm]
it	[ɪçt]	away from	[əweɪəfrʌm]
new dog	[nusdɔχk]	moving	[mufvĩ]
tell	[tsɛ]	deep	[dimp]
paste	[breɪs]	no good	[nou gʊd]
ball	[bwa]	zipper	[tzɪpɚ]
name	[neɪmp] [ndæ]	roof	[βupf]
my	[mbaɪ]	piece	[pitsi]
man	[mbænt]	bathroom	[bætərum]
toothpaste	[tuθpeɪs]	wish	[fwɪt]
everybody	[æfrtpɑdi]	we	[ɸwi]
cream	[tərim]	read	[vrid]

Exercise 1 Provide two examples of each of the following patterns of articulation in the table:

(a) insertion of a neutral vowel in a consonant cluster as the lips or tongue move too slowly to the next target
(b) insertion of a fricative during the formation or release of a stop
(c) insertion of a stop during the formation of a fricative
(d) insertion of a voiced or voiceless fricative during the formation of a glide
(e) insertion of a stop resulting from the raising of the velum during the release of a nasal sound

Exercise 2 The mistiming of laryngeal activity can result in devoicing of consonants in the productions in the table. Sometimes this occurs immediately prior to the production of the target voiced phoneme. Give one example of this pattern in the table.

Exercise 3 The deaf children studied by Smith sometimes came to a complete halt at syllable boundaries, represented by the insertion of a stop, before proceeding to the next syllable. Give two examples of this pattern of articulation in the data.

Exercise 4 During the release of bilabial stops, some of Smith's children continued to hold lip rounding after the constriction was released, resulting in the production of a glide. Give two examples of this articulation in the data.

Exercise 5 The mistiming of a particular articulatory movement led to the production of 'deep' as [dimp]. Which articulatory movement is responsible for this error?

9.4 Congenital hearing loss 2

Genetic syndromes are a significant cause of congenital hearing loss in children. Two such syndromes are branchio-oto-renal (BOR) syndrome and Stickler syndrome. The otological defects and hearing losses in these syndromes are described by Smith and Schwartz (1998) and Nowak (1998), respectively. Examine the clinical descriptors of these syndromes and then answer the questions below.

Branchio-oto-renal (BOR) syndrome

First described in 1975, BOR syndrome is an autosomal dominant disorder in which there is abnormal development of the first and second branchial arches. This results in a phenotype consisting of branchial, otological and renal defects. The disorder is rare – it has a prevalence of 1:40,000 on some estimates – but it is now recognized to be one of the more common forms of autosomal dominant syndromic hearing impairment. Among the common characteristics of the disorder are mild renal (kidney) anomalies, branchial fistulae, cup-shaped pinnae and preauricular pits. Other features include renal aplasia or agenesis, preauricular tags, lacrimal duct stenosis, a long, narrow face, deep overbite and a constricted palate.

There are significant ear anomalies and hearing loss in BOR syndrome. Preauricular pits, lop ear deformity and stenotic external auditory canals are found in approximately 80%, 35% and 30% of affected individuals, respectively. Other ear anomalies include ear canal atresia, ossicular defects (malformation, malposition, dislocation or fixation of the ossicles) and reduction in the size or malformation of the middle ear cavity. Cochlear hypoplasia is the most common inner ear problem, although enlargement of the cochlear and vestibular aqueducts and hypoplasia of the lateral semicircular canal are also found. Hearing loss is mixed in approximately 50% of individuals, but can also be conductive (approximately 25%) and sensorineural (approximately 25%) in nature. Hearing loss can range from mild to profound, and is severe in approximately 35% of cases. In about 25% of individuals, hearing loss is progressive.

Stickler syndrome

First described in 1965, Stickler syndrome is an autosomal dominant disorder which has, on some estimates, a prevalence of 1:10,000. An underlying abnormality in the collagen component of connective tissue results in defects in craniofacial, skeletal, ocular and auditory systems (collagen is a major component of the inner ear, for example). There are similar defects across systems. Alterations in the pigmented epithelium of the inner ear, for example, are akin to those found in the retina of the eye. Craniofacial and auditory anomalies are of most relevance to the speech-language pathologist. Individuals with Stickler syndrome have a flat facial profile with midface or mandibular hypoplasia. Facial asymmetry may also be present.

Micrognathia is a common feature, and the glossoptosis and cleft palate that is associated with the Robin sequence may also occur (a significant number of individuals with Robin sequence have been found to have Stickler syndrome on further investigation, as have clients with cleft palate). Clefts may affect the hard or soft palates, or both, are midline and posterior. A submucous cleft, bifid uvula, and a short or poorly mobile palate are more subtle palatal anomalies. The palatal defect is responsible for middle ear pathology in the form of recurrent otitis media with effusion, the latter necessitating the placement of ventilation tubes. Hearing loss may be pure conductive, pure sensorineural, or mixed, and is mostly mild to moderate.

Exercise 1 Conductive hearing loss is present in both syndromes. However, this loss is related to different ear anomalies. Describe the pathological mechanisms which cause conductive hearing loss in these syndromes.

Exercise 2 Sensorineural hearing loss is present in both syndromes. However, this loss is related to different ear anomalies. Describe the pathological mechanisms which cause sensorineural hearing loss in these syndromes.

Exercise 3 Only in BOR syndrome is hearing loss progressive in nature. The hearing loss in Stickler syndrome is generally no more progressive than that due to age-related hearing loss. Which pathological feature in BOR syndrome is believed to be responsible for progressive hearing loss?

Exercise 4 In both syndromes, there are pathological features which are normally contraindications for cochlear implants. Identify these features for each syndrome.

Exercise 5 Speech is likely to be hypernasal in only one of these syndromes. Identify the syndrome in question, and explain why hypernasality occurs.

9.4   Congenital hearing loss 3

The following case study is of a boy called George who was studied by Belenchia and McCardle (1985). George is 19 months of age and has Goldenhar's syndrome, a rare complex of symptoms which includes craniofacial and vertebral malformations. Examine the details of the case and then answer the questions below.

Medical history

George is the surviving child of a set of triplets. One sibling died of aspiration pneumonia at 17 days, and the other died of sudden infant death syndrome at 3 months. George was delivered by Caesarean section at 8 months gestation weighing 4lb 1oz. His 22-year-old mother had been under medical supervision for anaemia (iron deficiency) and toxaemia (pre-eclampsia) during pregnancy. There was no family history of either multiple births or congenital anomalies. At 5 months, George was diagnosed as having hydrocephalus which had arrested by 8 months, when he was readmitted to hospital with a fever and rash. A CT scan performed at this time revealed right frontal and temporal cortical atrophy, and cranial and facial asymmetry.

Developmental history

George's mother reported that he visually tracked objects at 6 months, reached for objects at 7 months, turned his head towards voices at 8 months and cooed at 10 months (the latter after lip repair).

Feeding

George experienced feeding difficulties due to his cleft lip, submucous cleft and gastroesophageal reflux. However, feeding had improved following lip repair and successful management of reflux.

Hearing

George has microtia and atresia of the right ear. An audiological assessment revealed that George responds to his name at 15 db HL, a 1500-Hz warbled tone at 20 db HL, and a bell at 30 db HL. Given George's atresia of the right ear, these levels are assumed to represent left ear performance.

Language

At 1 year, George underwent a speech-language evaluation. George's performance on two language assessments revealed a significant delay in overall language development, with performance at the 4–5 month age level on one assessment. Receptive language performance surpassed expressive language performance on both assessments – 6–7 months and 8 months for receptive language, and 2–3 months and 6 months for expressive language. At 19 months of age, and after 4 months of language therapy, George's language skills were re-evaluated. Tests revealed an overall language age of 20 months (one month above his chronological age), with a receptive language age of 26 months and an expressive language age of 21 months. On a further assessment, George had an auditory comprehension age of 30 months, and a verbal ability age of 20 months. He has appropriate pragmatic language skills, as evidenced by his ability to produce requests and comments and initiate communicative interactions.

Speech

George's speech is hypernasal with audible nasal emission due to velopharyngeal insufficiency. At 1 year, his vocalizations consisted of /ʌ/ with varied loudness, repetitive productions of /ŋʌ/ and, according to report, an occasional /m/ sound. During vocal play with his mother and the examiner, George did not attempt to imitate specific vowel or consonant sounds. Vocalizations were both random and in response to verbal stimulation. At 19 months, George had a repertoire of vowels and the consonants /k, g, ŋ n, b, m, w/.

Other skills

George displays age-appropriate functional play within the physical limitations of his syndrome (he has vertebral anomalies which include butterfly vertebral body in the mid-thoracic area with some cervical ribs). He also has some emerging motor imitation skills (e.g. he is able to wave bye-bye). Despite George's early developmental delays, mental retardation or intellectual disability is rare in Goldenhar's syndrome and, given George's rapid improvement in language skills as a result of therapy, is unlikely to be a significant factor in his case.

Exercise 1 George has unilateral microtia which affects his right ear. Which of the following statements is *true* of this ear anomaly?

(a) Unilateral microtia is about six times more frequent than bilateral microtia.
(b) Unilateral microtia is indicative of sensorineural hearing loss.
(c) Unilateral microtia is more common in males than in females.
(d) Unilateral microtia is always accompanied by preauricular pits and tags.
(e) Unilateral microtia is found predominantly on the right side.

Exercise 2 As George's case exemplifies, microtia is generally accompanied by hypoplasia of the ear canal. This ear canal abnormality can vary from a slightly narrowed canal to complete aural atresia. Explain why microtia and atresia frequently occur together.

Exercise 3 George's audiological assessment revealed hearing loss. What type(s) of hearing loss is this likely to be? Provide an explanation for your answer.

Exercise 4 George's speech is hypernasal with audible nasal emission on account of velopharyngeal insufficiency (VPI). The same palatal defect which gives rise to VPI also causes ear pathology. What is this pathology and what type of hearing loss is associated with it?

Exercise 5 At 1 year of age, George displays significant language delay. Which of the following factors is likely to make a significant contribution to this delay?

(a) George's intellectual skills
(b) George's speech delay
(c) George's social skills
(d) George's hearing loss
(e) George's motor skills

9.4   Congenital hearing loss 4

NC is a 10-year-old Dutch girl with Wolf-Hirschhorn syndrome who was studied by Van Borsel et al. (2004). This syndrome results from a distal deletion of the short arm of chromosome 4. The phenotypic expression, which is often severe, includes multiple malformations, delayed psychomotor development and profound learning disabilities. Examine the details of this case and then answer the questions below.

Medical history

NC is the oldest child of two healthy parents. Her younger sister is also healthy. During NC's prenatal development, there was intra-uterine growth retardation and birth weight, length and head circumference were all below normal (length and head circumference were on the 3rd centile, while birth weight was less than the 3rd centile). Features typical of Wolf-Hirschhorn syndrome were present at birth: cleft of the soft palate, a valvular pulmonal stenosis (a disorder that involves the pulmonary valve of the heart), renal tubal acidosis (a kidney abnormality which results in excessive acid in the blood) and hernia diaphragmatica (an abnormal opening in the diaphragm). High-resolution chromosomal analyses at 18 months confirmed the clinical diagnosis of Wolf-Hirschhorn syndrome. The terminal deletion of the short arm of chromosome 4 was confirmed by fluorescence in situ hybridization studies at 10;2 years.

Oral structure

The cleft of the soft palate was surgically repaired at 1;3 years. Crowding and an overbite were recorded during an orthodontic examination at 8;8 years. Ankylosis and poorly controlled tongue mobility were revealed in an ENT examination.

Hearing

Bilateral secretory otitis media was diagnosed at 4;10 years. At 8;9 years, pure tone audiometry revealed bilateral conductive hearing loss of 30 dB HL on average, which was more severe in the low frequencies.

Cognitive skills

NC had a total IQ of 55 at 4;11 years. A mean cognitive score below the 50th percentile and verbal and performance scale scores below the 22nd percentile were recorded during testing at 9;3 years.

Speech and language milestones

NC started to speak at around 4 years of age. She produced her first monosyllabic utterances and one-word sentences at 4;10 years. At that time, oral motoricity and phonological abilities were described as being limited. NC produced two-word sentences at 5;11 years, at which time articulation was reported to be markedly improved.

Language evaluation

NC's language skills were formally assessed on seven occasions between 3;3 and 9;8 years. Although receptive language skills were superior to expressive language skills, both were significantly below NC's chronological age. For example, at 6;6 years, NC's receptive and expressive language skills were commensurate with those of a child of 3;6 and 2;9–3;0 years, respectively. At 9;8 years, NC had the receptive language of a 4-year-old child, and the expressive language of a 3-year-old child.

Speech evaluation

NC received an extensive evaluation of her speech skills at 10;4 years. Voice quality and jitter and shimmer values were all judged to be normal. However, the fundamental frequency of NC's voice was significantly above average. NC displayed only mild hypernasality and no nasal emission, cul-de-sac resonance, assimilative nasality or nasal turbulence. These perceptual evaluations of nasality were confirmed by nasometry. NC's vowel inventory was almost complete, with only three Dutch vowels missing. Her consonant inventory was less complete, with 45.5% of consonants missing in prevocalic position, and 23.1% missing in postvocalic position. The overall percentage of vowels and consonants correct was 76.9% and 31.6%, respectively. By place of articulation, the consonants which were most often affected were the glottals, postalveolars, alveolars and velars. In terms of manner of articulation, liquids and fricatives were the most compromised. The following figures are the percentage of consonants correct in prevocalic position:

/z/ 0%	/f/ 87.5%	/m/ 81.8%
/v/ 7.7%	/s/ 20%	/n/ 50%

A phonological process analysis of NC's speech was also conducted. It revealed that cluster reduction and final consonant deletion were the most frequent syllable structure processes, while fronting and gliding were the most frequent substitution processes.

Exercise 1 NC exhibits mild hypernasality in her speech and has a conductive hearing loss. Which anatomical malformation in NC's phenotype explains these speech and hearing anomalies? Explain the causal mechanism in each case.

Exercise 2 Vowels are relatively spared in NC's speech, while consonants display a much greater level of impairment. How might this pattern be explained in terms of NC's hearing status?

Exercise 3 The consonants /z/ and /v/ are rarely, or never, correctly produced in prevocalic position, while another fricative sound /f/ has a much higher percentage of correct production in this position. Explain this pattern of consonant production in terms of NC's hearing loss.

Exercise 4 Despite both being high frequency fricative sounds, /f/ has a much higher percentage of correct production in prevocalic position than /s/. Which feature of the articulation of /f/ might make it an easier sound for NC to assimilate into her consonant inventory than /s/? Is this same feature able to explain any of the other patterns of consonant production displayed above?

Exercise 5 By place of articulation, the consonants which were most often affected in NC's speech were the glottals, postalveolars, alveolars and velars. Is there any other feature of NC's clinical presentation which may contribute to her difficulty in articulating alveolar sounds?

9.5   Sensorineural hearing loss 1

Background

The single-word productions below are from a boy of 6;1 years, known as Freddie, who was studied by Oller et al. (1978). Freddie was exposed to maternal rubella in the first trimester of pregnancy and has profound bilateral sensorineural hearing loss as a consequence.

Freddie's speech is characterized by phonological processes which are more typical of younger normal children, and normally hearing, language-delayed children.

Target word	Client production	Target word	Client production
skate	[kejt]	star	[ta]
keys	[ti]	dad	[da]
gun	[ɡʌn]	cracker	[ʈwáʈʊ]
shoe	[tu]	pencil	[pɛɳʈə]
zipper	[dɪpə]	house	[hawʈ]
radio	[weio]	brush	[bwʌtʂ]
blocks	[bwɔtʂ]	scissor	[ɖítə]
carrots	[teə]	lamb	[næm̃]
clock	[ka]	car	[ka]

Exercise 1 Freddie's single-word productions displayed a number of commonly occurring phonological processes. Four such processes are shown below. Provide two examples of each process in the above data:

(a) consonant cluster reduction
(b) final consonant deletion
(c) stopping
(d) liquid gliding

Exercise 2 Other phonological processes occurred less commonly in Freddie's speech. Two such processes are shown below. Provide one example of each process in the above data:

(a) deletion of medial liquid
(b) deletion of final liquid

Exercise 3 In what word positions does the process of stopping occur: word-initial, word-medial, or word-final position? Provide data to support your answer.

Exercise 4 Describe the phonological process at work in Freddie's production of 'lamb' as [næm̃].

Exercise 5 In prevocalic position, the liquids /l/ and /r/ are replaced by glides, e.g. blocks [bwɔtʂ] and brush [bwʌtʂ]. However, in postvocalic position liquids are replaced by mid and back vowels. Give two examples of this pattern in the data.

9.5 Sensorineural hearing loss 2

Meningitis is one of the most common causes of significant sensorineural hearing loss in children. The cases of three children with post-meningitic hearing loss, who were studied by Neuman et al. (1981), are described below. Examine the details of these cases and then answer the questions below.

Case A: Boy aged 5;9 years

Medical status

This boy was admitted to hospital with Haemophilus influenza type B. Purulent cerebrospinal fluid was obtained through lumbar puncture. Assessment revealed positive Brudzinski sign (flexion of the knees and hips in response to passive neck flexion) and a positive Kernig sign (an inability to extend the leg when the hip and knee are flexed). (Both signs are believed to result from irritation of motor nerve roots passing through inflamed meninges as the roots are brought under tension.) Positive blood and throat cultures were also obtained.

Hearing status

Three days after admission, the boy reported hearing loss. During an otological examination, both tympanic membranes were found to be slightly bluish in colour. A pure-tone assessment revealed total hearing loss in the left ear, and severe to profound, high-frequency sensorineural hearing loss in the right ear. The boy's fatigue prevented speech discrimination testing at the first session. Acoustic impedance measurements showed normal tympanograms bilaterally, but acoustic reflexes were absent. There was a significant improvement in hearing in the right ear at all frequencies, particularly the higher frequencies, approximately one month later. At this time, speech discrimination was 36%. Amplification and weekly speech and language therapy were commenced.

Six months later, there was no significant change in pure-tone thresholds in the right ear and no measurable hearing in the left ear. Speech discrimination was 36–60%. The right ear had a normal tympanogram, but there was negative H_2O pressure in the left ear. There was no acoustic reflex bilaterally. A myringotomy was performed along with placement of a pressure equalizing tube. Speech therapy continued on a weekly basis. There was still no measurable hearing in the left ear a year later. However, at this time, there was also a significant decrease in hearing sensitivity and speech discrimination in the right ear. Amplification was adjusted to accommodate these poorer thresholds, and speech and language therapy was increased. There was still a normal tympanogram in the right ear and negative pressure in the left ear. A normal tympanogram was subsequently achieved in the left ear.

Case B: Boy aged 3;6 years

This boy was hospitalized with meningococcal meningitis. Hearing loss was not reported during treatment. However, the family reported a significant change in hearing ten days after treatment. Initially, audiological evaluation revealed total hearing loss in the right ear and moderately severe sensorineural hearing loss in the left ear. Both ears showed significant negative pressure on acoustic impedance measurements. With the exception of a left-ear reflex at 500 Hz (120 dB HL), acoustic reflexes were absent bilaterally. An otolaryngologist recommended medication to treat the middle ear problem. Amplification and twice-weekly language stimulation were instituted. Some eight months later, when the boy was seen again, pure-tone thresholds were 10–20 dB poorer in the left ear. The total hearing loss in the right ear was unchanged. A normal tympanogram was obtained for the left ear, but acoustic impedance measurements revealed significant negative pressure in the right ear. There was no further change in hearing at a later audiological evaluation.

Case C: Boy aged 2;9 years

This boy was hospitalized with Haemophilus influenza type B meningitis. EEG tracings and otological examinations were normal on admission. An audiological evaluation was conducted one month after discharge because the child's parents had noticed a hearing problem. It revealed a bilateral, moderately severe to profound, sloping sensorineural hearing loss. Acoustic reflexes were absent bilaterally but tympanograms were normal. Amplification with a hearing aid was instituted. Approximately three months later, a re-evaluation showed hearing to be stable in the left ear and a significant improvement in hearing in the right ear at 500, 1000 and 2000 Hz. Amplification with a different aid and therapy continued. One month later, a further significant improvement in hearing was noted. Acoustic reflexes were present bilaterally at 500 and 1000 Hz. At this time, there was a marked improvement in speech and language therapy tasks. Over two years later, thresholds in the right ear were stable through 2000 Hz, while there was a significant decrement (no measurable hearing) at 4000 and 8000 Hz. Acoustic reflexes were absent bilaterally. Acoustic impedance measurements revealed negative pressure in the right ear. The boy's progress is good with his present amplification.

Exercise 1 On the basis of the above cases, which of the following statements characterize hearing loss in post-meningitic paediatric patients?

(a) High frequencies are more adversely affected than low frequencies.
(b) Hearing loss may be asymmetrical.
(c) A central auditory processing disorder is a consistent feature.
(d) When hearing fluctuations occur, they can be quite significant in extent.
(e) When changes in children's hearing level are observed, they generally occur in the lower frequencies.

Exercise 2 Do any of these children exhibit middle ear pathology? Provide evidence to support your answer.

Exercise 3 Which of the following procedures conducted in these children is/are sensitive to the presence of cochlear pathology?

(a) electroencephalography (EEG)
(b) tympanometry
(c) acoustic reflex test
(d) lumbar puncture
(e) myringotomy

Exercise 4 An otolaryngologist recommended medication to treat the middle ear problem of the boy in Case B. What is this middle ear problem likely to be and what form might this child's medication take? Is there any evidence that the recommended treatment has been effective? Provide evidence to support your answer.

Exercise 5 The child in Case C experiences significant improvement in his hearing in the right ear at 500–2000 Hz, and a significant decrement at 4000 and 8000 Hz. What is the likely effect of this pattern of hearing loss on this child's recognition of English vowels and consonants?

9.6   Cochlear implantation 1

Background

Speech intelligibility was examined in 20 paediatric users of cochlear implants studied by Chin et al. (2001). All children had profound bilateral hearing losses. They had all experienced onset of deafness before 3 years of age, had been fitted with a cochlear implant before 6 years of age and had been using an implant for at least two years. The chronological age of the children at the time of testing ranged from 4;8 to 7;8 years. Two intelligibility tests used minimal pairs to assess the perception and production of sound contrasts. Some of these pairs are shown below.

bat–pat	two–shoe	beet–boot	van–fan
feet–fat	fell–shell	bear–pear	pill–pool
boot–boat	pie–tie	big–bug	bomb–mom
bat–mat	pat–fat	pat–cat	goat–coat
pea–key	leaf–laugh	pea–paw	bee–boo

Prosodic and voice anomalies have also been observed in children with hearing loss. These anomalies have been found in children with and without cochlear implants. The prosodic and voice characteristics of six children with cochlear implants were examined by Lenden and Flipsen (2007) during conversational speech. The chronological age of children at the start of the study was 3;9 to 6;2 years. All children were prelingually deaf and had been fitted with a cochlear implant by 3 years. At the onset of testing, all children had used cochlear implants for at least 18 months. The following table shows the number of conversational samples for these children in which at least 90% of coded utterances were judged to be appropriate (pass), 80–90% of coded utterances were judged to be appropriate (borderline) and less than 80% of coded utterances were judged to be appropriate (fail) for seven prosody and voice variables.

Variable	Pass	Borderline	Fail
Phrasing	36	4	0
Rate	22	13	5
Stress	2	5	33
Loudness	32	2	6
Pitch	38	2	0
Laryngeal quality	24	7	9
Resonance quality	0	1	39

Exercise 1 Using the minimal pairs in the first table above, give one example of a pair for each of the following contrasts:

(a) *Vowel height*: High vs. low
(b) *Place of articulation*: Labiodental vs. alveopalatal
(c) *Voicing*: Voiced bilabial vs. voiceless bilabial
(d) *Manner of articulation*: Oral vs. nasal
(e) *Vowel backness*: Front vs. back

Exercise 2 Which contrast is exemplified by the minimal pairs in (a) below? Some minimal pairs in (b) contain segments that differ by a single phonetic feature, while others contain segments that differ by two phonetic features. For each pair under (b), indicate the number of phonetic features (one or two) and type of phonetic features (voicing, place of articulation, etc.) that are involved in the contrast.

(a) van–fan; two–shoe; pea–key; boot–boat; goat–coat; pie–tie
(b) bear–pear; pat–fat; pea–paw; pat–cat; two–shoe

Exercise 3 There were no significant correlations between any of the five pairs of feature classes – vowel height, place of articulation, voicing, manner of articulation and vowel backness – in the minimal pairs perception and production tests. What does this finding suggest about the remediation of speech perception and production skills in children with cochlear implants?

Exercise 4 The second table above records the performance of six children along a number of prosody and voice variables. Stress and resonance quality are the two most deviant variables in these children. These variables were also found to be significantly correlated with post-implantation age (amount of implant use). What do these correlations reveal?

Exercise 5 For resonance quality, 89.8% of the inappropriate utterances were coded as being 'nasopharyngeal'. Describe this pattern of resonation in these children.

9.6   Cochlear implantation 2

Amplification by means of a hearing aid may not provide a child with sufficient auditory stimulation to ensure the development of central auditory pathways. In such cases, cochlear implantation may be indicated. Dorman et al. (2007) argue that the latency of the P1 component of the cortical evoked response to sound may serve as a biomarker for maturation of central auditory pathways and, as such, can function as an indicator of when cochlear implantation becomes necessary. The P1 response is 'generated by auditory thalamic and cortical sources' and its latency 'reflects the accumulated sum of delays in synaptic propagation through the peripheral and central auditory pathways' (2007: 285). Dorman et al. demonstrate the clinical value of the P1 component by means of the following case studies. Examine the details of these cases and then answer the questions below.

Case A

This patient, a female child, had a normal birth history. However, she failed newborn hearing screening and, at 2 weeks, auditory brainstem response testing revealed a bilateral, severe-to-profound hearing loss. It emerged upon further testing that congenital cytomegalovirus was a likely cause of the child's hearing loss. At 5 months of age, she was fitted with a hearing aid. The unaided pure-tone average for the right ear when tested in soundfield was 100 dB. The left ear exhibited no response at any frequency. A pure-tone average of 78 dB HL was obtained in soundfield testing using binaural hearing aids. Cortical auditory evoked potentials were recorded after seven months of hearing aid use in an aided soundfield. At the maximum equipment output levels, a P1 response could not be detected. Standard criteria for cochlear implantation were met by the patient, and at 19 months of age a cochlear implant was fitted in her right ear. Over the next four months, the P1 latency decreased by 200 milliseconds. The P1 latency at four months was within normal limits and remained so when testing occurred at seven months after implantation. The patient also displayed progress in speech and language acquisition.

Case B

This patient, a male child, failed newborn hearing screening and was diagnosed with hearing loss. A severe-to-profound hearing loss was diagnosed when he was 5 months of age using auditory brainstem response testing. The child's hearing loss was secondary to Goldenhar's syndrome. He also presented with microtia and atresia of the right ear and its canal. At 9 months of age, he was fitted with a hearing aid in the left ear. However, soundfield testing revealed no aided benefit in the left ear, and behavioural audiometric testing confirmed severe-to-profound hearing loss in the left ear and profound hearing loss in the right ear. At 17 months after the fitting of his hearing aid, cortical auditory evoked potentials testing was conducted in an aided soundfield setting. At the maximum output levels of the equipment, no P1 response could be elicited. The patient satisfied standard criteria for cochlear implantation and, at 2;7 years of age, a cochlear implant was fitted in his left ear. At the time of implant hookup and at 6 and 13 months post-implantation, further cortical auditory evoked potentials recordings were made. At hookup, P1 latency was significantly delayed and remained prolonged at 6 and 13 months post-implantation. These findings suggested that there had been a lack of normal central auditory pathway development. They were also consistent with the audiologist's observation that the child was behaviourally unresponsive to auditory stimuli and did not wear his cochlear implant with consistency.

Exercise 1 The child in Case A displayed no P1 response when tested after using a hearing aid for seven months. What is the significance of this finding?

Exercise 2 The child in Case A only received a cochlear implant in her right ear when, in fact, she had a bilateral sensorineural hearing loss. Why might this be the case?

Exercise 3 The child in Case B had a cochlear implant in his left ear only. Why would an implant of the right ear be contraindicated in this particular child? What type of hearing loss is associated with the conditions you identified in your response to the last question?

Exercise 4 The hearing of the child in Case B is examined using behavioural and physiological tests. Why should both types of test be used in paediatric audiometry?

Exercise 5 The latency of the P1 response following implantation decreased markedly in the child in Case A but remained prolonged in the child in Case B. How would you explain this difference?

SUGGESTIONS FOR FURTHER READING

Ackley, R. S. 2014. 'Hearing disorders', in L. Cummings (ed.), *Cambridge handbook of communication disorders*, Cambridge: Cambridge University Press, 359–80.

Alexiades, G., De La Asuncion, M., Hoffman, R. A., Kooper, R., Madell, J. R., Markoff, L. B., Parisier, S. C. and Sislian, N. 2008. 'Cochlear implants for infants and children', in J. R. Madell and C. Flexer (eds.), *Pediatric audiology: diagnosis, technology, and management*, New York: Thieme, 183–91.

Fuller, D. R., Pimentel, J. T. and Peregoy, B. M. 2012. *Applied anatomy and physiology for speech-language pathology and audiology*, Baltimore, MD and Philadelphia: Lippincott Williams & Wilkins (chapter 13).

Haynes, W. O., Moran, M. J. and Pindzola, R. H. 2012. *Communication disorders in educational and medical settings: an introduction for speech-language pathologists, educators and health professionals*, Sudbury, MA: Jones & Bartlett (chapter 10).

Humes, L. E. and Bess, F. H. 2008. *Audiology and communication disorders: an overview*, London and Philadelphia: Lippincott Williams & Wilkins (chapter 4).

Møller, A. R. 2012. *Hearing: anatomy, physiology, and disorders of the auditory system*, San Diego, CA: Plural Publishing (chapter 9).

Peterson-Falzone, S. J., Hardin-Jones, M. A. and Karnell, M. P. 2010. *Cleft palate speech*, St. Louis, MO: Mosby Elsevier (chapter 6).

Pratt, S. R. and Tye-Murray, N. 2009. 'Speech impairment secondary to hearing loss', in M. R. McNeil (ed.), *Clinical management of sensorimotor speech disorders*, second edition, New York: Thieme, 204–34.

Stach, B. A. 2010. *Clinical audiology: an introduction*, second edition, Clifton Park, NY: Delmar (chapters 3 and 4).

Stach, B. A. and Ramachandran, V. S. 2008. 'Hearing disorders in children', in J. R. Madell and C. Flexer (eds.), *Pediatric audiology: diagnosis, technology, and management*, New York: Thieme, 3–12.

Answers to questions and exercises

Chapter 1: Introduction to communication disorders

1.1 Human communication and its disorders

(1) intention. (2) part (b). (3) False. (4) part (a). (5) False. (6) part (a). (7) part (c). (8) part (b). (9) True. (10) part (d).

1.2 Significant distinctions in speech-language pathology

(1) part (c). (2) True. (3) False. (4) parts (b), (c) and (d). (5) parts (a) and (d). (6) acquired; fragile; developmental; gestation; traumatic; adulthood; language; execution; velopharyngeal; palate; palsy; syntactic; voice; aphasia; intellectual; expressive; receptive; encoding; passive. (7) parts (a), (b) and (e). (8) parts (b), (d) and (e). (9) False. (10) True.

1.3 Disciplines integral to speech-language pathology

(1) part (b). (2) part (c). (3) parts (b), (d) and (e). (4) True. (5) False. (6) parts (b) and (c). (7) endocrinologist. (8) psychologist. (9) psychiatrists. (10) pragmatics.

1.4 Human communication breakdown

(1) language encoding. (2) language encoding; language decoding; motor execution. (3) communicative intentions. (4) motor execution. (5) sensory processing. (6) motor programming.

1.5 Clinical distinctions

(1) The term 'acquired' in *acquired* epileptic aphasia relates to the fact that a significant amount of language acquisition has taken place prior to the onset of Landau-Kleffner syndrome. (2) Patrick's problems with syntax are receptive in nature. His difficulties with semantics are expressive. (3) Penelope has a speech disorder. (4) John has receptive and expressive pragmatic problems. (5) Frank's grammatical delay is developmental, while his dysarthria is acquired. (6) Paul has a language disorder.

1.6   Foundational disciplines

Part A: Linguistics

(1) syntax. **(2)** phonology. **(3)** pragmatics. **(4)** semantics. **(5)** morphology. **(6)** phonetics. **(7)** discourse. **(8)** phonology. **(9)** pragmatics. **(10)** syntax.

Part B: Medicine

(1) anatomy. **(2)** otorhinolaryngology. **(3)** physiology. **(4)** embryology. **(5)** neurology. **(6)** anatomy. **(7)** psychiatry. **(8)** genetics. **(9)** neurology. **(10)** otorhinolaryngology.

Chapter 2: Developmental speech disorders

Section A: Short-answer questions

2.1   Cleft lip and palate

(1) velum; plosives; nasal; grimacing; glottis; glottal; dental; fistulae; speech; vocal; hearing; conductive; Eustachian; veli; middle; otitis media; equalizing; tympanic; myringotomy; amplification. **(2)** parts (a), (c) and (d). **(3)** part (c). **(4)** False. **(5)** True. **(6)** part (a). **(7)** part (c). **(8)** palatoplasty. **(9)** phonology. **(10)** True.

2.2   Developmental dysarthria

(1) traumatic brain injury; meningitis; postnatal; palsy; cerebrovascular accidents; dystrophy; fossa; cranial; facial; lesion; upper; spastic; ataxic; phonation; velopharyngeal; nasal; instrumental. **(2)** parts (b) and (d). **(3)** parts (a), (c), (d) and (e). **(4)** prenatal. **(5)** prosody. **(6)** part (a). **(7)** parts (a), (b), (d) and (e). **(8)** parts (b), (c) and (d). **(9)** False. **(10)** False.

2.3   Developmental verbal dyspraxia

(1) part (d). **(2)** False. **(3)** True. **(4)** True. **(5)** True. **(6)** parts (a), (b) and (d). **(7)** parts (a), (c) and (e). **(8)** decrease. **(9)** part (c). **(10)** part (c).

Section B: Data analysis exercises

2.4   Cleft lip and palate 1

Exercise 1 The hypernasality and nasal emission in Louise's speech is most likely to be related to the presence of a submucous cleft palate. However, given that Louise also exhibits some hypotonia, the involvement of neurological factors as well as structural problems cannot be discounted in this articulatory deviance. **Exercise 2** (a) Frication. (b) Stopping. (c) Fronting. (d) Backing. 'kruis': frication; 'kop': fronting. **Exercise 3** (a) /siˠaRɛt/ → [sizaRɛt]. (b) /fits/ → [sis]. (c) /ˠitər/ → [Ritə]. (d) /wɔlkən/ → [wɔk]. (e) /jɔŋən/ → [ɔŋə]. **Exercise 4** (a) /kr/ undergoes cluster reduction in 'tap' and frication in 'cross'. (b) /rst/ is reduced to /s/ in 'sausages' and to /t/ in 'brush'. (c) /ən/

is deleted in 'clouds' and reduced to /ə/ in 'boy'. (d) /k/ undergoes fronting in 'head' and frication in 'clock'. In short, there is considerable variability in Louise's speech production with one and the same target being differently realized on separate occasions. **Exercise 5** (a) cluster reduction and syllable deletion. (b) cluster reduction and syllable deletion. (c) initial and final consonant deletion.

2.4   Cleft lip and palate 2

Exercise 1 Rachel does observe the phonotactic structure of targets. Rachel marks each element in the target with a corresponding segment, even though the latter is phonetically distant from the target form, e.g. 'glasses' /ˈglæsɪz/ CCVCVC → [ˈɴwæ̥ɕə̥ɕ] CCVCVC. Rachel signals a contrast between the alveolar nasal /n/ and the alveolar plosives /t/ and /d/ through the use of a uvular nasal /ɴ/ and glottal plosive /ʔ/, respectively. The velar nasal /ŋ/ and velar plosives /k/ and /g/ are similarly contrasted. **Exercise 2** The bilabial nasal /m/ is consistently correct in Rachel's speech. The bilabial plosives /p/ and /b/ are variously realized in Rachel's speech: /p/ → [ʘ], [ʔ], [ʘ͡ʔ], [p̚ʔ]; /b/ → [m], [ɓ], [b]. Only rarely does Rachel achieve full oral status for bilabial plosives, and even then only in the case of /b/. However, despite the variability of these realizations, some of which have nasal involvement, Rachel is still able to maintain a rudimentary oral–nasal contrast in her production of bilabial sounds. **Exercise 3** The approximants /j/ and /w/ are correctly realized in Rachel's speech. Stops are realized word-initially by the glottal plosive [ʔ]. Alveolar fricatives /s/ and /z/ and the postalveolar fricative /ʃ/ are consistently realized in word-initial position as [ɕ̯]. So Rachel does have an effective articulatory strategy for signalling a contrast between stop, fricative and approximant sounds. The stop–affricate contrast is realized in word-initial position by [ʔ] and [ʔj], respectively. Rachel separately marks the stop and fricative elements in an affricate. Once again, although her productions are phonetically distant from the target in each case, she is nevertheless able to signal a contrast between stops and affricates. **Exercise 4** Rachel's alveolar and postalveolar fricatives are consistently realized as [ɕ̯]. So although she is no longer using pharyngeal articulations for these sounds, she has still not succeeded in consistently signalling an alveolar–postalveolar contrast during the production of fricatives. However, Rachel does display a habitual tendency to labialize the postalveolar fricative /ʃ/ which may indicate an attempt on her part to signal an alveolar–postalveolar contrast. **Exercise 5** The voicing contrast is marked for the bilabial plosives /p/ and /b/. However, there is no voicing contrast observed for the alveolar plosives /t/ and /d/ or the velar plosives /k/ and /g/, all of which are realized as [ʔ]. Rachel variously signals a voicing contrast between /f/ and /v/. On some occasions, she uses the approximant [ʋ] for /v/ (e.g. 'cover'). On other occasions, a voicing distinction is marked by differing forces of articulation with /v/ realized as [f] in contrast with the weakly articulated [f̬].

2.5   Developmental dysarthria

Exercise 1 Cluster reduction: 'brush' [bəʂ]; 'smoke' [moːʔʂ]; palatoalveolar fronting: 'sugar' [ʂəʂə]; 'brush' [bəʂ]; velar fronting: 'sock' [ʂɒʔʂ]; 'sugar' [ʂəʂə]. Palatoalveolar fronting occurs in all positions. For example, there is fronting of /ʃ/ word-initially in 'sugar' and word-finally in 'brush', and fronting of /tʃ/ word-medially in 'matches'. Velar fronting only occurs in non-initial positions. For example, there is fronting of /g/ word-medially in 'sugar' and fronting of /k/ word-finally in 'sock'. However, velar fronting occurs inconsistently in word-final position, as is illustrated by 'milk' where /k/ is not fronted. **Exercise 2** Alveolar fricatives are realized with a slit articulation [ʂ] rather than the grooved articulation that is the adult form. Mike uses [f] for dental fricatives in word-initial position (e.g. 'three') and [ʂ] for these fricatives in other positions (e.g. 'nothing', 'teeth'). **Exercise 3** (a) [ɸ] in 'penny'; [ʂ] in 'cotton'; [ʂ] in 'boat'. (b) [ʂ] is used in place of /tʃ/ in 'chimney', 'matches' and 'watch'. The pattern is stopping. **Exercise 4** The production of /k/ as [ʂ] involves both fronting (a velar sound is realized as an alveolar sound) and the use of a slit rather than a grooved articulation. **Exercise 5** Aspiration of voiceless plosives in word-initial position: [pʰ] in 'paper'; [tʰ] in 'teeth'; [kʰ] in 'cat'. Three realizations of voiceless plosives and affricates: (a) aspiration (e.g. [pʰ] in 'paper'); (b) affrication (the realization of plosives as homorganic affricates, e.g. [ts] in 'tea'); (c) spirantization (the realization of plosives and affricates as homorganic fricatives, e.g. [ʂ] in 'chimney').

2.6 Developmental verbal dyspraxia

Exercise 1 Repeated tokens of 'cat' and 'plate' display segmental variability. The variability in the production of 'cat' occurs on the vowel sound (/æ/ and /ɛ/). The variability in the production of 'plate' affects the word-initial cluster /pl/ and the word-final consonant /t/. **Exercise 2** 'Dog' and 'chair' do not display the token variability evident in 'cat' and 'plate'. Even as the speaker is unable to produce the target for 'chair', the erroneous tokens do not display variability. **Exercise 3** rain /weɪn/ liquid gliding; girl /dal/ fronting; bridge /wedʒ/ consonant cluster reduction; liquid gliding. **Exercise 4** On the basis of Data 2, Ryan's sound substitutions would appear to be consistent. For example, word-initial /k/ is consistently fronted to [d] in 'kangaroo' and 'cake'. The liquid /r/ is consistently glided to [w] in 'rain' and 'bridge'. **Exercise 5** Ryan is able to produce diphthongs such as /eɪ/ in 'cake' and 'rain', and /aɪ/ in 'dinosaur'.

Chapter 3: Developmental language disorders

Section A: Short-answer questions

3.1 Developmental phonological disorder

(1) part (a). **(2)** part (d). **(3)** True. **(4)** False. **(5)** True. **(6)** part (c). **(7)** vowel. **(8)** stimulable. **(9)** parts (a), (b) and (d). **(10)** True.

3.2 Specific language impairment

(1) parts (c) and (d). **(2)** aetiology; hearing; specific; syntax; inflectional; auxiliary; object; semantic; pragmatics; secondary. **(3)** True. **(4)** False. **(5)** pronoun; auxiliary. **(6)** tense. **(7)** parts (a), (b), (d) and (e). **(8)** part (a). **(9)** True. **(10)** 1.25; 85.

3.3 Developmental dyslexia

(1) parts (a), (b), (c) and (e). **(2)** False. **(3)** parts (c) and (e). **(4)** orthographic; spelling; automatic; developmental; writing; dysgraphia; oral. **(5)** parts (b), (c), (d) and (e). **(6)** False. **(7)** True. **(8)** English has a highly opaque orthography in comparison to other languages (e.g. German). That is, the connection between graphemes and phonemes is not straightforward, with the same sound written in different ways (e.g. photography, finish) and the same letter or combination of letters standing for different sounds (e.g. church, chasm). **(9)** parts (a), (c) and (e). **(10)** True.

3.4 Intellectual disability

(1) part (d). **(2)** parts (b) and (d). **(3)** parts (a) and (c). **(4)** foetal alcohol syndrome. **(5)** True. **(6)** True. **(7)** False. **(8)** parts (a), (b), (c) and (e). **(9)** False. **(10)** Down's syndrome.

3.5 Autism spectrum disorder

(1) pervasive; pragmatic; conversation; turns; force; prosodic; facial; cognition; mental states; question; request. **(2)** False. **(3)** True. **(4)** True. **(5)** parts (b) and (d). **(6)** parts (d) and (e). **(7)** parts (a) and (c). **(8)** False. **(9)** false belief. **(10)** True.

3.6 Childhood traumatic brain injury

(1) True. **(2)** False. **(3)** intact; white; axonal; haemorrhages; bony; frontal; oedema; haematoma; open; metabolic; subtle; mismanagement; phonology; syntax; recover; pragmatics; traumatic. **(4)** parts (a), (b), (d) and (e). **(5)** parts (b) and (c). **(6)** True. **(7)** True. **(8)** semantic. **(9)** part (b). **(10)** cognitive.

3.7 Landau-Kleffner syndrome

(1) parts (a) and (c). **(2)** Landau; onset; epileptiform; rare; prevalence; residential schools; more; insidiously; secondary; auditory agnosia; normal; hyperactivity; cognitive; stuttering. **(3)** True. **(4)** False. **(5)** part (c). **(6)** parts (a), (c) and (e). **(7)** True. **(8)** True. **(9)** few. **(10)** parts (a), (c) and (d).

Section B: Data analysis exercises

3.8 Developmental phonological disorder 1

Exercise 1 /ʃ/ and /ʒ/ are realized as [ʧ] and [ʤ], respectively. These realizations occur before the vowels [a] and [u] in syllable-initial within word position. **Exercise 2** /ʃ/ and /ʒ/ are differently realized in (8) to (10). These sounds are both realized as [t]. It is clear from these productions that /ʃ/ and /ʒ/ are realized as [t] in syllable-initial word-initial position. **Exercise 3** This pattern of realization is not maintained in (11) to (15). In these productions, /ʃ/ and /ʒ/ are both realized as [t]. **Exercise 4** In (11) to (15), /ʃ/ and /ʒ/ are realized as [t] because they occur in a stressed syllable. The general rule that captures the pattern of realization of /ʃ/ and /ʒ/ across (1) to (15) can be stated as follows: /ʃ/ and /ʒ/ are realized as [ʧ] and [ʤ] *unless* they occur in syllable-initial word-initial position (in which case they are realized as [t]), and *unless* they occur in a stressed syllable (in which case they are realized as [t]). In other words, the [ʧ] and [ʤ] realizations are only found when /ʃ/ and /ʒ/ occur in syllable-initial within word position and in an unstressed syllable. **Exercise 5** In (16) to (21), there is velar fronting of /k/ and /g/ to [t] and [d], respectively. The fact that [t] and [d] in the single-word productions in (19) to (21) are not replaced by [ʧ] and [ʤ], as we would expect them to be based on the pattern identified in Exercise 4, is an indication that velar fronting is a completely separate process in D's phonological system. So we end up with [atí] and not [aʧí] as we would expect, given that [t] is occurring in syllable-initial within word position and in a stressed syllable.

3.8   Developmental phonological disorder 2

Exercise 1 Consonant cluster reduction: /plato/ → [lato]; /krus/ → [tus]. Liquid simplification: /plato/ → [pato] (omission of liquid); /plato/ → [pwato] (gliding of liquid). **Exercise 2** Velar fronting: /krus/ → [tlus]; /krus/ → [tus]. Velar fronting only occurs in the context of word-initial consonant clusters. When /k/ occurs as a singleton both in word-initial and word-medial positions, it is not fronted, e.g. /kasa/ → [kaθa]; /boka/ → [βoka]. **Exercise 3** Deaffrication: /ʧina/ → [ʃina]. Backing: /raton/ → [ʀakon]. Denasalization: /mansana/ → [pasan]. **Exercise 4** matíta 'pencil' [tita]; martéllo 'hammer' [telo]; caróta 'carrot' [rota]. **Exercise 5** Deletion of word-medial weak syllables in: álbero 'tree' [albo]; pécora 'sheep' [peka]; péttine 'comb' [pete].

3.8   Developmental phonological disorder 3

Exercise 1 (a) fish [vɪ]; class [gæ]; (b) bag [bæ]; web [wɛ]; (c) vegetables ['vɛbɛ]; probably ['pwɒ.bɪ]. **Exercise 2** light [jaɪ] gliding; queen [ki:] consonant cluster reduction; sink [dɪ] stopping. **Exercise 3** final consonant deletion; consonant cluster reduction; prevocalic voicing. **Exercise 4** Final consonant deletion: bag [bæ] pre-intervention; [bæg] post-intervention. Prevocalic voicing: pram [bæ] pre-intervention; [pæm] post-intervention. **Exercise 5** (a) horse [ɔ:t]; sitting ['dɪ.tə]. (b) stairs [dɛə]; try [daɪ]. (c) fell [fɔ:n]; down [dãu].

3.9   Specific language impairment 1

Exercise 1 (a) 'He eating'. (b) 'Her painting'. (c) 'She building block'. (d) 'He's marrying my dad'. (e) 'Why he fall in the car?'. **Exercise 2** SLI children of the same chronological age are making different grammatical errors. For example, of the two children who are 4;2 years, one is using a subject pronoun when needed (albeit the incorrect subject pronoun), while the other child is still using the object pronoun, i.e. 'And her painting now' and 'He's marrying my dad'. This same pattern is also seen in the two children who are 4;10 years. **Exercise 3** Possessive pronouns, e.g. 'He kinda has a hat like yours'. **Exercise 4** (a) False: noun phrases are used with premodifiers in 'a hat', 'the car', and 'my dad'. (b) False: the inflectional suffix *-ing* is used on all main verbs where it is required. (c) False: these children are also using prepositional phrases (e.g. 'in the car') and adverb phrases (e.g. 'right here'). (d) True: examples are 'Her's painting a flower' and 'He's marrying my dad'. (e) True: the verb 'is' appears as an auxiliary in 'He's marrying my dad' and as a main verb in 'He's a cop'. **Exercise 5** More mature grammatical forms are not consistently found in the older children with SLI. For example, a child of 4;10 years is still using an object pronoun rather than a subject pronoun ('Her's painting a flower'), while a younger child of 4;1 years is using the correct subject pronoun ('Yeah, he sleeping right here').

3.9 Specific language impairment 2

Exercise 1 (a) 'I just fall down on my bike'. (b) 'I flied and then I jumped down'. (c) 'I went to um Toys "Я" Us and gave me a toy' (implicit 'I' subject is incorrect). (d) 'I jumped out of my bike'. (e) 'everybody was sad that um uh that died' (subject pronoun 'she' to refer to grandmother is omitted). **Exercise 2** (a) Extract 1: 'they're checking on my leg'. (b) Extract 1: 'I was going up there'. (c) Extract 1: 'My ma and dad went to the funeral and then Aunt Cindy was there too and we uh they . . .' (does 'they' refer to Aunt Cindy as well as mum and dad, or to just mum and dad?). (d) Extract 2: 'went to the park'. (e) Extract 2: 'It was not a long way to get to the hotel. We went to a hotel' (the indefinite noun phrase 'a hotel' should precede the definite noun phrase 'the hotel'). **Exercise 3** The boy in Extract 1 has the worse topic management skills. He fails to develop a topic to any extent before leaving it for another topic and then eventually returning to the original topic. For example, the topics in R's first extended turn in Extract 1 can be represented as follows: leg – toys – leg – bike. In R's second extended turn in Extract 1, his topic structure appears as follows: bike accident – death of grandmother – funeral – bike. **Exercise 4** In Extract 2, there is considerable repetition concerning the distance to locations, the hotel and keys. Repetitive language conveys no new information and thus frustrates the development of a story during narrative production. **Exercise 5** In Extract 1, R states: 'I did it with uh I did do it with only my hands. I didn't do it without my hands'. In Extract 2, L states: 'It was a long way to get there [. . .] it was a short way [. . .] it was not a long way to get to the hotel'. In Extract 2, L also says that dad gave the keys to the girl who then gave the door keys to the door. This type of illogicality makes the narrative difficult to comprehend.

3.9 Specific language impairment 3

Exercise 1 Utterances (a), (c), (d), (g), (h), (i) and (l). **Exercise 2** The use of the infinitive 'to go' is impaired in utterance (b) but is intact in utterance (e). MM produces an inflected infinitival complement in (b) with 'to' omitted as well. In utterance (k) there is another example of an inflected infinitival complement with 'to' omitted. **Exercise 3** In utterances (m) and (n), subordinate conjunctions 'if' and 'when' are used for the first time. In utterance (m), there is a single subordinate conjunction clause (if you just shoot it) followed by a coordinate conjunction clause (and it makes a basket). In utterance (n), there are two subordinate conjunction clauses (if you're bouncing it when you're walking it). **Exercise 4** Utterance (f): omission of the obligatory complementizer 'if' in a full propositional clause. Utterance (j): omission of obligatory relative marker 'who'. Utterance (o): omission of the complement-taking verb 'say' or 'tell' for the WH clause. **Exercise 5** Utterance (a): the people → people. Utterance (e): a long way → long ways. Utterance (m): a point → a points.

3.10 Developmental dyslexia

Exercise 1 (a) e.g. metamorphosis [mɛtapoɯrʌs]; grotesque [grɔtikə]. (b) e.g. fascinate 'fascinated'. (c) e.g. adventurously 'adventurous'. (d) e.g. pivot 'pirate'; systematic 'sympathetic'. **Exercise 2** JR is attempting to identify word subcomponents in the target (e.g. 'incontinental') rather than sound out the target grapheme by grapheme. **Exercise 3** The errors in Data 3 are neologistic in nature. JR is using visual segmentation skills to identify words within the target (e.g. 'disportionately'). However, the fact that he is able to read *dis-* (similarly, *cir-* of the non-word 'cirsemicular') shows that he is also using phonological skills to read words and non-words. **Exercise 4** (a) False: while 'ritual' may well be a low-frequency word in English, 'friend' is certainly not. (b) False: errors affect concrete words (e.g. leopard) and abstract words (e.g. honour). (c) False: vowel letters are also affected as in menace → maness, and trouble → troble. (d) True: examples are prairie → prair (omission of letters 'ie'), and health → heath (omission of letter 'l'). (e) False: all JR's written spelling errors conform to orthographic rules of English. **Exercise 5** Yes.

3.11 Intellectual disability 1

Exercise 1 Stopping, e.g. /s/ → [t] in 'gnome', 'backpack' and 'teddy bear'. Devoicing, e.g. /b/ → [p] in 'car', 'ball' and 'teddy bear'. Final consonant deletion, e.g. deletion of /ɭ/, /n/ and /l/ in 'car', 'water' and 'ball', respectively. **Exercise 2** An epenthetic vowel is used in each of these productions, i.e. /ɔ/ in 'flower' and 'blue', and /ə/ in 'apple' and 'snake'. **Exercise 3** The glottal fricative [h] replaces oral sounds in 'draw', 'bird' and 'shower'. The two sound classes affected by this substitution are the plosives /t/ and /d/, and the fricative /f/. **Exercise 4** The nasal sounds /n/ and /m/ are omitted in 'window' and 'teddy bear', respectively. The lateral approximant /l/ and /ɭ/ is omitted in 'ball' and 'car', respectively. **Exercise 5** (a) False: she omits all consonants in her production of 'crown' as ['ʉæ]. (b) True: she fails to produce /kʰ/ and /tʰ/ in 'clock' and 'roof', respectively. (c) True: the final consonant in /'nø.kɭ/ becomes the first consonant in ['lɒŋ.æ]. (d) False: /s/ → [θ] in 'light'. (e) True: /ʊ/ → [m] in 'water' and /b/ → [ʊ] in 'battery'.

3.11 Intellectual disability 2

Exercise 1 Pronouns (e.g. it, they); verbs (e.g. go, have); nouns (e.g. dog, puppy); determiners (e.g. a); most notably, there are no adjectives, adverbs, prepositions or conjunctions. **Exercise 2** There is evidence of morphological immaturity in JB's omission of the inflectional suffix *-es* in 'it go woof woof'. **Exercise 3** Lexical immaturity is suggested by JB's use of the onomatopoeic form 'woof woof' instead of the verb 'bark'. **Exercise 4** JB omits the genitive form 's (e.g. 'uncle bed'); JB omits the preposition 'in' (e.g. 'I go sleep [in] uncle room'); JB omits the conjunction 'and' (e.g. 'I go [and] sleep . . . '); JB omits the possessive determiner 'my' (e.g. 'I go sleep [my] uncle room'). **Exercise 5** (a) True: JB uses a range of gestures quite effectively to support his spoken language. (b) True: JB is talking around the target words in each of these utterances. (c) True: the presence of circumlocution suggests that JB has word-finding problems. (d) False: JB is able to convey his message quite effectively through a combination of linguistic and gestural skills. (e) True: when JB is making a request to push the equipment cart for one last time in (1), he uses the term 'please'.

3.11 Intellectual disability 3

Exercise 1 (a) /bl/ → [b] in 'black'; /fl/ → [f] in 'flower'. (b) deletion of /n/ in 'gun'; deletion of /z/ in 'nose'. (c) /g/ → [t] in 'gun'; /g/ → [d] in 'green'. (d) /v/ → [b] in 'vase'; /ð/ → [d] in 'that'. (e) /dʒ/ → [ʧ] in 'page'; /v/ → [f] in 'glove'. **Exercise 2**

(a) /s/ deletion; consonant cluster reduction; consonant cluster deletion. (b) /θ/ deletion; liquid gliding; final consonant deletion. (c) depalatalization; consonant cluster deletion; liquid gliding; final consonant deletion. (d) /l/ deletion; stopping; syllable deletion. (e) initial consonant deletion; /s/ deletion; voicing; final consonant deletion. **Exercise 3** (a) 'flower' and 'music box'. (b) 'gun' and 'green'. (c) 'sweater' and 'flower'. (d) 'sled' and 'truck'. (e) 'feather' and 'vase'. **Exercise 4** (a) False: there is still velar fronting at 4;7 years, e.g. /k/ → [d] in 'Ken'. (b) False: there is still stopping at 4;7 years, e.g. /f/ → [d] in 'foot'. (c) True: word-final /k/ is present in 'cheek' but not in 'duck'. (d) True: at 4;0 years 'farm' is produced as [mɑm]. (e) True: 'duck' and 'dog' are both produced as [də]. **Exercise 5** There is evidence of monopthongization of dipththongs at both 4;0 and 4;7 years in the production of 'goat'.

3.11 Intellectual disability 4

Exercise 1 (a) /pl/ and /tr/. (b) /mp/; /tl/; /rf/ and /rst/. (c) /nt/; /ft/ and /ts/. **Exercise 2** (a) Liquid deviation; other examples: ['moːlən] → ['moːrən]; [baˈlɔn] → [baˈrɔŋ]; ['taːfəl] → ['taːfər]. (b) Deletion of unstressed syllables; other example: [ˌkaˈbɔutər] → ['bɔutəʳ]. (c) Backing of alveolar plosives; other examples: [dri] → [kri]; [trap] → [krap]. **Exercise 3** Consonant harmony: ['pɔtloːt] → ['pɔploːt]; [brɪl] → [blɪl]. Vowel-consonant harmony: ['pɔtloːt] → ['pɔkloːt]; ['trɔməl] → ['tlɔŋər]. **Exercise 4** (a) ['zeːvən] → [seːvŋ]; ['eːzəl] → ['eːsəl]; [ˌkaˈbɔuter] → [ˌkaˈpultər]. (b) [ˌʃoːkoːˈlaːdə] → [soːkəˈlaːdə]; [ʒiˈraf] → [ʑiˈraf]. (c) [baˈlɔŋ] → [pəˈrɔŋk]; [plasˈtrɔŋ] → [pasᵗˈrɔŋk]; [ˌtɪfəˈfɔŋ] → [ˌtɪləˈfɔŋk]. **Exercise 5** (a) Partial reduplication. (b) Voicing of intervocalic consonants. (c) Coalescence. (d) Metathesis.

3.12 Autism spectrum disorders 1

Exercise 1 'his back' (whose back?), 'that boy' (what boy?), 'the man' (what man?), 'they got' (who got?). The problem with referring expressions indicates that the boy is not able to appreciate the knowledge state of his listener (the examiner). The listener has no referents for these expressions, a fact which is not grasped by the boy in Extract 1. He is unable to establish the knowledge state of the examiner on account of a weakness in ToM. **Exercise 2** part (c). **Exercise 3** This boy is unable to attribute to the mother the communicative intention that motivated her utterance, namely, that the mother is stating that the girl is wearing her best clothes with a view to urging her to keep them clean. **Exercise 4** Egocentric discourse is also evident in Extract 2 when the boy utters 'I always have fun when I climb up a tree'. Egocentricity in discourse reveals a failure on the part of the speaker to assume the perspective of the listener. In the absence of this perspective, the egocentric speaker dominates the verbal interaction with topics and experiences which are not of interest or relevance to the listener. **Exercise 5** The boy in extract 2.

3.12 Autism spectrum disorders 2

Exercise 1 (a) /k/ → [t] 'cow'; /k/ → [d] 'sky'. (b) /f/ → [b] and /ʃ/ → [t] 'fish'. (c) Deletion of /v/ in 'glove'; deletion of /n/ in 'green'. (d) /k/ → [d] 'sky'; /t/ → [d] 'tub'. (e) /sp/ → [b] 'spoon'; /sn/ → [z] 'snail'. **Exercise 2** (a) Final consonant deletion; stopping; prevocalic voicing. (b) /s/ cluster reduction; fronting; prevocalic voicing. (c) Final consonant deletion; consonant cluster reduction; liquid gliding. **Exercise 3** 'snail', 'sled' and 'snake' realized as [zʌ]; 'tub' and 'thumb' realized as [dʌ]; 'spring' and 'three' realized as [ɰi]. **Exercise 4** Stops: 'butter' [bʌʔə]; 'sleeping' [ɰiʔi]. Liquids: 'squirrel' [ɰəʔə]; 'jelly' [dzʌʔi]. **Exercise 5** 'horse' [haω], 'jelly' [dzʌʔi], 'book' [bʌ], 'snail' [zʌ].

3.12 Autism spectrum disorders 3

Exercise 1 In Extracts 1 and 2, Helen is repeating the final word(s) of a speaker's prior turn – 'mountain' (Extract 1) and 'way sign' (Extract 2). This behaviour, known as immediate echolalia, is commonly found in autism. **Exercise 2** In these same extracts, Helen also repeats the word(s) she repeated from the speaker's prior turn. This further repetition, known as palilalia, is a repetition of an initiating word(s) within Helen's own utterance rather than a final word within another speaker's utterance. **Exercise 3** Helen's first attempt to provide an answer to Nigel's numerical problem is effectively overlooked by him. Helen's response was somewhat mistimed, as she came in with a response too early – the teacher Nigel intended to elicit a somewhat formulaic response to the problem which involved the answer 'number eight'. By repeating her response, Helen is ensuring that it is acknowledged by Nigel in a way that her single-word response was not. **Exercise 4** In Extracts 1 to 3, Helen's repetitions are serving as some form of response to a speaker's prior turn – a question (Extract 1), a directive (Extract 2) and a numerical problem (Extract 3). In Extract 4, Helen is using repetition not as a response to a prior turn, but as an initiating action, in this case a request. **Exercise 5** In Extract 5, Helen is using repetition concurrently with an action, the transfer of a block to Nigel's hand. Each use of the word 'three' in this repetition corresponds to a particular stage in this action. Helen is able to terminate her repetition of 'three' with the completion of the action, suggesting that her repetition is an attempt to frame her non-vocal activities in this exchange.

3.13 Childhood traumatic brain injury

Exercise 1 (a) 'Ummm, I, once, there was a, we went'. (b) 'all kinds of stuff there'. (c) Discussion of cat: 'She has a cat named Gus, a kitten. It's so cute'. (d) 'And one day, I have a friend named Jude' (this temporal expression is incongruent with the introduction of a friend). (e) The child gives a detailed account of where she was stung, then talks about the medical assistance she received at her friend's house, and returns to discuss further where she was stung. **Exercise 2** (a) 'I have a friend named Jude. She's umm grown up' (anaphoric reference). (b) 'my cousin Matt got stung in one of the private parts. And umm I had a bite right here' (collocation). (c) 'The bees chased us and I looked back. And there was one right in front of my face' (substitution). **Exercise 3** (a) False: the child uses fillers such as 'umm' extensively, which may suggest some word-finding difficulties. But her pointing gestures are not related to word-finding difficulties. (b) False: the narrative is difficult to follow, but not on account of any grammatical difficulties. (c) True: this is evident when she introduces the fort, then leaves it to talk about a tree and dirt, and then returns to the fort. (d) True: she starts her narrative with the expression 'once', and attempts to set the scene for the listener through utterances like 'There was this fort'. (e) False: there is no clear evidence of semantic paraphasias in this narrative. The word 'bite' *may* be a semantic paraphasic error (target 'sting'). **Exercise 4** (a) The child explicitly introduces characters and agents into the narrative and then refers to them through pronominal reference (e.g. 'She has a cat named Gus, a kitten. It's so cute').

Through doing so, she ensures that the listener can track the various protagonists in the story. (b) The child ensures that her listener knows the referents of adverbs such as 'here' and 'there' by pointing to specific body parts. (c) The child expends considerable effort introducing the familial and other relationships she has with each of the characters in the story (e.g. my cousin Matt, my brother Jason, my friend Jude). Some of these are stated on more than one occasion during the narrative. This indicates an attempt on the part of the child to give the listener some background knowledge within which to process the details of the narrative. **Exercise 5** Quantity: too much information is conveyed in parts, such as the excessively detailed explanation of where each of her friends was stung. Relation: the child veers off topic and begins to talk about irrelevant points such as her friend's kitten. Manner: some information is confusing, ambiguous and contradictory, such as when we are told about the topical medication that the child received. First, we are told 'I put it on me'. Then, we are told 'she [Jude] put it on me'. Finally, we are told 'I had to go to the bathroom to put it on'.

3.14 Landau-Kleffner syndrome

Exercise 1 The two conditions – one suspected, the other diagnosed – which were credited with explaining Dillon's symptoms were hearing loss and pervasive developmental disorder. Even though these conditions were ultimately shown to be mistaken, they were at least consistent with many of the behaviours Dillon was displaying. Hearing loss was suggested by the fact that Dillon did not respond to his name being called in class. His lack of response to direct attempts to engage him might also suggest hearing loss. Of course, what appeared to be hearing loss was, in fact, the auditory agnosia of Landau-Kleffner syndrome. Dillon's normal audiological evaluation revealed that he heard what people were saying, but did not recognize their spoken words. Pervasive developmental disorder was also suggested by Dillon's behaviours. Dillon's poor social skills with both his peers and adults were consistent with the socialization impairment of pervasive developmental disorder. A severe regression in skills, such as Dillon experienced, is also indicative of pervasive developmental disorders. Aside from Dillon's marked social and communication impairments, he also exhibited some problems with fine motor skills, another feature of pervasive developmental disorders. **Exercise 2** Standardized language tests are assessing structural language skills (e.g. syntax, semantics). However, in order to use language in communication with others, Dillon needs to draw on pragmatic language skills. These latter language skills are rarely assessed by standardized language tests. So Dillon's structural language skills are relatively intact at 4;1 years, while his use of language (pragmatics) in communicative situations is impaired. This explains the disparity between Dillon's good test performance and the impaired communication skills which Dillon's teachers are observing. **Exercise 3** parts (b), (c) and (d). **Exercise 4** Dillon has cognitive deficits in the areas of attention and executive function. That there is cognitive involvement in some of Dillon's expressive language problems is suggested by his request for more pizza and by his response to winning the board game. Dillon's request for a bigger piece of pizza suggests that he is not satisfied with the size of the piece he has currently. His subsequent acceptance of this piece indicates that he has lost sight of the goal which motivated his original request. This failure of goal-directed behaviour is consistent with Dillon's difficulties with executive function. Dillon also appears to have, at best, a fleeting memory of having won the board game he was playing with his mother and sister. This may suggest a problem with short-term memory or, alternatively, a failure to attend properly to the result of the game (a failure of attention). **Exercise 5** parts (d) and (e).

Chapter 4: Communication disorders in mental illness

Section A: Short-answer questions

4.1 Schizophrenia

(**1**) mental illness; equal; earlier; morphology; phonology; inflectional; derivational; object; subordinating; neologisms; perseveration; pragmatics; speech acts; conversational; quantity; relation. (**2**) parts (a) and (e). (**3**) True. (**4**) False. (**5**) True. (**6**) part (b). (**7**) part (c). (**8**) *Diagnostic and Statistical Manual of Mental Disorders.* (**9**) delusions; alogia (poverty of speech). (**10**) cohesion.

4.2 Bipolar disorder

(**1**) manic; normal. (**2**) psychomotor. (**3**) False. (**4**) part (c). (**5**) parts (b), (c) and (d). (**6**) mania; manic-depressive illness; euthymia; hypomania; depression; mania; remission; tangentiality; rapid; hypomanic; topical; pressured. (**7**) False. (**8**) False. (**9**) True. (**10**) sound.

4.3 Emotional and behavioural disorders

(**1**) part (c). (**2**) parts (a), (b) and (c). (**3**) False. (**4**) True. (**5**) True. (**6**) True. (**7**) behavioural; *Diagnostic and Statistical Manual of Mental Disorders*; hyperactivity; impulsivity; inattention; excessive; answers; listen; interrupt; social communication. (**8**) parts (a), (b) and (d). (**9**) parts (b) and (e). (**10**) externalizing.

Section B: Data analysis exercises

4.4 Schizophrenia 1

Exercise 1 noosle → noose + nozzle; rath → raft + wreath; captus → cactus + octopus (also, /p/ from octopus and /t/ from cactus); octatoos → octopus + cactus. **Exercise 2** cactus: 'the thing you find in Mexico'; abacus: 'math beads, math scale'. **Exercise 3** sound and functional features: 'microscope' for *telescope*; visual relationship: 'bubble' for *rattle*; 'microscope' for *telescope*. **Exercise 4** On some occasions, phonemic cues are effective in eliciting the target (e.g. 'rattle'), while on other occasions they are not (e.g. 'abacus'). **Exercise 5** Use of 'Christmas' for stimulus item *wreath*; use of 'rope' for stimulus item *noose*; use of 'abstract' for stimulus item *maze*.

4.4 Schizophrenia 2

Exercise 1 The client reveals an appreciation of narrative structure through the use of an introduction to the story, i.e. 'I was watching a film of a little girl . . . ' **Exercise 2**

'little girl ... she just went to the store ... ' (anaphoric reference); 'her brother ... he was blamed ... ' (anaphoric reference). **Exercise 3** Egocentric discourse emerges early in the narrative at the point of 'bring back memories of things that happened to uh people around me that affected me during the time when I was living in that area ... '
Exercise 4 The client is using a range of expressions during egocentric discourse which do not relate to the ice cream story and for which no clear referent can be identified, e.g. 'I was living in that area ... ' and 'I'm kinda like asking could we just get together ... '
Exercise 5 Cohesion is achieved through the underlined words: 'bring back memories of things that happened to uh people around me that affected me during the time when I was living in that area ... '

4.4   Schizophrenia 3

Exercise 1 Morphological errors: use of 'medicate' instead of 'medicat-*ion*' (omission of derivational morpheme); use of 'help' instead of 'help-*ed*' (omission of inflectional morpheme); use of 'memory' instead of 'memor-*ize*' (omission of derivational morpheme). These morphological errors could be somewhat differently construed as errors in the selection of words from particular grammatical classes. In this way, the use of 'medicate' instead of 'medication' could be construed as the erroneous selection of a verb instead of a noun. Also, the use of 'memory' instead of 'memorize' could be construed as the erroneous selection of a noun instead of a verb. **Exercise 2** There is evidence of perseveration in this extract: 'you should be able to ... you should be able to ... you should be able to ... '; 'with the food and medicate the food and medicate and the the food an medicate ... '; **Exercise 3** Compound nouns: thought process; thought pattern; mental process; brain wave; memory knowledge. **Exercise 4** This client is able (a) to use verbs in the active voice and the passive voice (e.g. 'I still do not have this' and 'I am being helped') and (b) to use modal auxiliary verbs (e.g. 'you *should* be able to'). This client is unable (a) to use auxiliary verbs on all occasions when they are required (e.g. 'I still not have the thought pattern') and (b) to use the infinitive form of the verb in all instances when it is required (e.g. 'you should be able to *memory* all the knowledge'). **Exercise 5** The following features are suggestive of a word-finding difficulty: (a) the presence of non-specific vocabulary (e.g. 'I still do not have *this*'); (b) repetition followed by filler and non-specific vocabulary (e.g. 'and the an the ah rest ... '); (c) reformulation which contains lexical items semantically related to target (e.g. 'the old te- the old *new* testament ... ').

4.4   Schizophrenia 4

Exercise 1 In the pre-intervention interview, lengthy pauses consistently occur at the end of PQ's utterances. Normally, even the smallest pauses at the end of an utterance lead to the exchange of turns between the participants in a conversation. The doctor delays assuming the turn from PQ as he is trying to encourage him to develop further his minimal response. It is only after a substantial pause when it is apparent that PQ is not going to do this that the doctor assumes the turn from PQ. In the post-intervention interview, pauses are less frequent and much shorter than in the pre-intervention interview. This is because PQ's much fuller responses satisfy the doctor's need to be given a certain amount of information with the result that the doctor more readily assumes the turn from PQ. **Exercise 2** The following linguistic features are infrequently used:

verbs – only five main verbs (relax, get, be, think, improved) are used by PQ in the whole interview; pronouns – PQ only uses the personal pronoun 'I' twice throughout the entire interview. There are many occasions when it is demanded but omitted (e.g. 'could be a bit better'). Although it is difficult to say with certainty why these features occur infrequently, their lack of use is likely to be related to PQ's general passivity in communication and low self-esteem. Specifically, the pronoun 'I' places PQ in the role of an agent who is responsible for the actions of verbs. By omitting this pronoun and verbs, PQ is able to remove agency from himself when he feels unable or unwilling to undertake actions. Adverbs are particularly common in the pre-intervention interview. Many of these adverbs express doubt and uncertainty on the part of PQ (e.g. *possibly* at night). Other adverbs and expressions serve to diminish or qualify what PQ is saying (e.g. *Bit of* salivation *occasionally*). **Exercise 3** The following linguistic features are present in the post-intervention interview: personal pronouns (e.g. I, she, her) are used extensively; use of proper nouns for names of people (e.g. Mary, Sally); main verbs are used throughout the interview; addresses the doctor by saying 'hello' (no greeting used in the pre-intervention interview). The improved self-evaluative status of PQ post-intervention may explain the presence of these linguistic features. Specifically, PQ appears more willing post-intervention to discuss his activities (achieved through the use of verbs) and significant others in his life (the presence of names) than he was pre-intervention. Also, there is greater awareness of the need to attend to social functions in communication (hence, the use of a greeting). **Exercise 4** In the pre-intervention interview, PQ merely responds to questions and never asks questions. On several occasions during the post-intervention interview, PQ poses questions to the doctor. These differences are likely to reflect a move away from a passive style of communication pre-intervention to a more assertive communication style post-intervention in which PQ feels motivated to ask questions and assume more control in the interaction. In the post-intervention interview, for example, PQ does not just use questions to gain information and clarification (e.g. Do I just walk in?) but also to query why something is happening (e.g. Why Tuesday? Why has it changed?). **Exercise 5** In the pre-intervention interview, PQ allows the doctor to frame the topic of discussion entirely by posing all the questions in the exchange. There is no attempt on PQ's part to either initiate a topic or develop in any way one of the topics introduced by the doctor. In the post-intervention interview, PQ provides more expansive answers which are serving to develop the topics under discussion. For example, the topic of PQ's leave was developed to include who he stayed with, who drove him to his destination and a fairly detailed list of the activities which were undertaken while he was away. The question 'When are you seeing X?' would have received a minimal response of 'Tomorrow' in the pre-intervention interview. However, in the post-intervention interview PQ adds that the community psychiatric nurse is changing jobs and will be replaced by a new person. Also in the post-intervention interview, PQ shows for the first time a willingness to develop topics in ways that are of interest to him by asking questions that address his specific informational needs (e.g. How often do I go?).

4.5　Bipolar disorder

Exercise 1 The speaker in Data 2 displays poverty of speech. He or she uses single-word responses (e.g. right) or short phrases (e.g. it could be) with no further elaboration. Such elaboration is necessary given that the interviewer is posing open questions to the depressed speaker. **Exercise 2** The speaker in Data 1 is making excessive use of negative utterances. Three examples of this behaviour are 'I just didn't feel', 'I didn't want to run', and 'I wouldn't let her'. **Exercise 3** The speaker in Data 3 makes excessive use of verbs of mitigation to reduce commitment to the truth of claims. Two examples of this behaviour are 'I could talk to you' and 'people seem friendly'. The repeated use of 'you know' – it is used four times – indicates a desire on the part of the depressed speaker to receive reassurance from his listener. **Exercise 4** The patient's yellow shirt appears to trigger the image of the US born, spiritual figure Baba Ram Dass ('it reminds me . . . '). There may be a visual similarity between the patient's shirt and attire worn by Ram Dass, and this may have triggered the patient to talk about him. **Exercise 5** The sounds in the Buddhist chant 'ohm ohm' are reversed to form 'mo'. The patient links the sound sequence 'mo' to the letters MO which act as a semantic trigger for the patient to talk about the US state of Missouri. Having mentioned Missouri, the patient then develops another sound association between the chant 'ohm' and the name of a bar in town called 'omni'. In the same way that he reversed the sounds in the chant to form 'mo', the patient then reverses the letters in the name of the bar to form INMO. The initial letters in this sequence then serve as a semantic trigger for him to name another US state, this time Indiana. A final sound and/or letter association may trigger the patient to utter 'universe' instead of 'United States'.

4.6   Emotional and behavioural disorders

Exercise 1 Abraham: 'bestest' (incorrect inflectional suffix); 'I throw the ball' (non-finite verb instead of past tense (finite) verb); 'he throw the pillow in my face' (non-finite verb instead of past tense (finite) verb); Adam: 'a hooks' (indefinite article with plural noun); 'you got hold' (use of 'got' instead of 'get'). **Exercise 2** (a) False: both children comprehend the teacher's questions with no evidence of difficulty. (b) True: both children exchange turns with the teacher at appropriate junctures. (c) True: even Adam's extended turn is not excessively lengthy given that it is a response to an open question from the teacher. (d) False: Abraham develops humour which is age-appropriate for his audience. (e) True: Adam's first turn contains repetitive language. **Exercise 3** Adam's extended turn is difficult to follow because he makes use of referring expressions without first establishing referents for those expressions. Examples include: 'they have a machine' (who has a machine?); 'he spins you' (who spins you?); 'they have a little round thing' (who or what has a little round thing?). **Exercise 4** The expressions 'then' and 'and then' are used by these children to extend their turns. Adam uses 'and then' no less than five times in his extended turn with the teacher. For the language impaired child, this simple linguistic expression permits the continuation of a turn in the absence of a more sophisticated repertoire of language and pragmatic skills. Its use permits the child speaker to add further clauses and hold the conversational floor while doing so. **Exercise 5** These children are desirable interlocutors for a number of reasons. Firstly, Adam is able to select a topic which is of interest to his same-age peers (i.e. snow tubing). Secondly, Abraham recounts a scenario with his baby brother that most young children would find humorous and appealing. Thirdly, it is likely that both children have an energetic and enthusiastic style of delivery – most likely related to their impulsive, hyperactive behaviour – which would also appeal to others. This is in stark contrast to the reticence of many children of 7;10 years (the age of Adam at the time of the study).

Chapter 5: Acquired speech disorders

Section A: Short-answer questions

5.1 Glossectomy

(1) squamous cell. **(2)** compensations. **(3)** part (a). **(4)** mobility; amount. **(5)** parts (a), (b) and (d). **(6)** False. **(7)** True. **(8)** True. **(9)** part (e). **(10)** part (b).

5.2 Acquired dysarthria

(1) head injury; neurodegenerative; neurone disease; worsen; treatment; progressive; alternative; cognitive; production; velopharyngeal; respiratory; articulatory; plosives; palatal. **(2)** parts (c) and (d). **(3)** part (c). **(4)** False. **(5)** True. **(6)** parts (b) and (c). **(7)** part (c). **(8)** (a) substantia nigra; (b) cerebellum; (c) demyelination; (d) motor cortex; (e) surgery. **(9)** parts (b) and (c). **(10)** parts (a), (c) and (e).

5.3 Apraxia of speech

(1) parts (b) and (d). **(2)** programming; dysarthria; neurological; automatic; length; groping; vowels; aphasia; differential. **(3)** parts (b) and (d). **(4)** parts (a) and (b). **(5)** True. **(6)** False. **(7)** True. **(8)** parts (a) and (c). **(9)** perception; increasing; multiple; instrumental; rate; duration; consonant; larynx; velopharyngeal; acoustic; diagnosis; onset. **(10)** parts (c) and (d).

Section B: Data analysis exercises

5.4 Glossectomy

Exercise 1 The plosive sounds /t, d/ are replaced by glottal stops (e.g. /t/→[ʔ] in 'stritten') and bilabial stops (e.g. /t/→[p] in 'stärkeren'). These substitutions have compensatory qualities. The speaker who is unable to use the tongue to achieve closure at the alveolar ridge for /t/ uses a glottal place of articulation instead (blockage of the pulmonary airstream at the glottis is possible). Similarly, [p] is used in place of /t/, because the bilabial plosive achieves the required blockage of the airstream when an alveolar place of articulation is not possible. **Exercise 2** The voiceless velar plosive /k/ is replaced by the voiceless velar fricative (e.g. /k/→[x] in 'daherkam'), while the voiced velar plosive /g/ is replaced by the voiced velar fricative (e.g. /g/→[ɣ] in 'gehüllt'). The patient who cannot elevate the back of the tongue to make contact with the velum in order to produce the velar plosives /k/ and /g/ approximates this articulation by using the velar fricatives [x] and [ɣ], respectively. The voiceless velar plosive is also replaced by uvular fricatives. This can be seen in /k/→[χ] in 'stärkere' and /k/→[ʁ] in 'stärkeren'. This retracted pattern of articulation is explained by Barry and Timmermann (1985) as follows. The speaker who produces one of these substitutions had one third of the tongue removed. The remaining part of the tongue was sewn to the floor of the mouth. The fixed tongue body made palatal contact impossible. Back closures were consequently shifted back to a point where the mandibular-maxillar angle provided natural proximity of the tongue and soft palate. As a result, uvular sounds came to substitute velar sounds. **Exercise 3** The substitution /d/→[s] in 'daherkam' contains the following three articulatory features: (a) lack of closure for plosive resulting in a fricative, (b) the loss of voicing, and (c) the lost voicing seems to be displaced onto the voiceless glottal fricative producing its voiced counterpart (i.e. /h/→[ɦ]). **Exercise 4** Consonant clusters that contain /t/ are either reduced (/ʃtʁ/→[ʁ] in 'stritten') or /t/ in these clusters is replaced by a bilabial plosive (/ʃt/→[ʃp] in 'stärkeren'). The difficulty with the alveolar place of articulation extends beyond plosives to include nasals with /n/→[m] in 'warmen'. Once again, a bilabial articulation is taking the place of alveolar articulation in the patient with compromised lingual movement. **Exercise 5** (a) /ʃ/ → [f] a labiodental fricative takes the place of a palato-alveolar fricative. (b) /ç/→[θ], a dental fricative replaces a palatal fricative. The mobility of the tongue tip makes dental friction possible where palatal friction could not be achieved on account of the relative immobility of the tongue body.

5.5 Acquired dysarthria 1

Exercise 1 The two phonetic features present in the first production of 'questions' but absent in the second production are: (a) a lack of frication at the end of the first syllable of 'questions' which is repaired by the speaker in the second production of this word; (b) the hypernasality that is present in the first production of 'questions' is not present in the second production of this word. **Exercise 2** There is zero closure at the end of the word 'fast' with no final plosive produced [fæs]. The complete closure that is needed to produce the alveolar plosive /t/ of 'too' is not achieved. Rather, during the production of [s̺] the tongue advances towards this closure without actually achieving it. **Exercise 3** (a) pit–pet. (b) bea–pea. (c) sip–ship. (d) dot–knot. (e) high–eye. (f) spit–pit. **Exercise 4** Stop–fricative: tip–sip; /r/–/w/: row–woe. **Exercise 5** Initial cluster-null phonetic contrast.

5.5 Acquired dysarthria 2

Exercise 1 parts (a), (b) and (e). **Exercise 2** Atrophy of the palate is a bulbar sign. Spastic weakness of the lips and tongue is a suprabulbar sign. **Exercise 3** The neuromuscular deficit ataxia results in the incoordination of movements across phonation, resonation and articulation. Hypotonia causes muscular weakness which results in the reduced range and force of movement. **Exercise 4** parts (a) and (b). **Exercise 5** (a) True, (b) False, (c) True, (d) False, (e) True.

5.5 Acquired dysarthria 3

Exercise 1 parts (a), (c) and (d). **Exercise 2** (a) The production of word-final consonants was particularly difficult for R. (b) Early treatment focussed on increasing R's vocal volume. Later treatment also emphasized adequate respiratory support for speech. It is clear from these various interventions that respiration was compromised for R. (c) R exhibited velopharyngeal dysfunction and speech hypernasality. (d) R's reduced vocal volume may be indicative of inefficient glottal valving of the pulmonary airstream. (e) Treatment targeted more effective use of stress and intonation patterns, suggesting both must be problematic for R. **Exercise 3** Slowed rate of speech had a significant, beneficial effect on the intelligibility of R's speech, because the reduction in rate gave the articulators more time in which to move to their targets. Syllable-by-syllable production also enhanced speech intelligibility. However, this was achieved by manipulating the prosodic features of speech. Specifically, during this compensatory technique, each syllable is produced with equal stress and duration. These prosodic adjustments, which are often employed as natural compensatory techniques by both dysarthric and dyspraxic speakers, serve to increase articulatory accuracy and the coordination of speech production subsystems (e.g. respiration and phonation). **Exercise 4** parts (b), (d) and (e). **Exercise 5** R's medical management and speech intervention were repeatedly compromised by behavioural issues which were related to his poor psychiatric status. R failed to comply with his medical regimen following diagnosis, which led to a worsening of his neurological condition. R was also unwilling to make adjustments to his daily routine in order to ensure that he received enough sleep to be able to comply with speech intervention. We are not told if R experienced psychiatric problems prior to the onset of Wilson's disease at 23 years of age. So problems of this nature may well be a premorbid characteristic of R. But what can be said with certainty is that psychiatric illness is commonly associated with Wilson's disease. Shanmugiah et al. (2008) examined psychiatric comorbidities in 50 confirmed patients with Wilson's disease and found that 12 patients (24%) fulfilled diagnostic criteria for a psychiatric diagnosis. Among these psychiatric diagnoses were bipolar affective disorder, major depression (a significant problem in R's case) and dysthymia.

5.6   Apraxia of speech

Exercise 1 (a) metathesis. (b) anticipatory. (c) reiterative. (d) anticipatory. (e) reiterative. (f) metathesis. (g) anticipatory. **Exercise 2** (a) Feature (2) – Exhibits phonemic perseverative errors. (b) Feature (5) – Exhibits phonemic vowel errors. (c) Feature (1) – Exhibits phonemic anticipatory errors. (d) Feature (1) – Exhibits phonemic anticipatory errors. (e) Feature (4) – Exhibits phonemic voicing errors. **Exercise 3** This speaker displays inconsistency of errors (Feature 8) with 'chookun' and 'dook' used in place of the target 'cushion'. The speaker has also produced a phonemic transposition error (Feature 3) which involves reversal of the positions of /k/ and /ʃ/ of 'cushion'. **Exercise 4** This speech behaviour shows that the speaker is aware of his error even as he is unable to correct it (Dabul's Feature 14). **Exercise 5** In 'patastrofee', the speaker achieves the last three syllables of the target form. However, in 'katasrifrobee', the speaker achieves the first two syllables of the target form. So there is inconsistency in D.B.'s production of syllables.

Chapter 6: Acquired language disorders

Section A: Short-answer questions

6.1   Acquired aphasia

(1) non-fluent; Wernicke's; expressive; agrammatic; comprehension; conversation; aware; semantic; unaware; neologisms; jargon; preserved; circumlocution; perseveration. **(2)** False. **(3)** True. **(4)** False. **(5)** parts (b) and (e). **(6)** parts (a), (c) and (e). **(7)** left. **(8)** written. **(9)** parts (c) and (e). **(10)** parts (a), (b) and (d).

6.2 Right-hemisphere language disorder

(**1**) parts (b) and (d). (**2**) aphasias; pragmatics. (**3**) part (c). (**4**) language; inadequately; concrete; questions; information; inferences; topic; pragmatics. (**5**) False. (**6**) True. (**7**) True. (**8**) part (d). (**9**) intentions. (**10**) False.

6.3 Traumatic brain injury

(**1**) True. (**2**) True. (**3**) part (b). (**4**) frontal. (**5**) executive; mind. (**6**) False. (**7**) False. (**8**) parts (a), (c) and (e). (**9**) intentions. (**10**) part (e).

6.4 Dementias

(**1**) part (c). (**2**) True. (**3**) True. (**4**) False. (**5**) part (b). (**6**) parts (a), (b) and (c). (**7**) augmentative; alternative. (**8**) semantic; phonology. (**9**) False. (**10**) True.

Section B: Data analysis exercises

6.5 Acquired aphasia 1

Exercise 1 Phonemic paraphasias: rubber-rudder; cope-coop. Semantic paraphasias: 'car' instead of truck or lorry; 'money' for food. **Exercise 2** Hesitations, e.g. 'he got th-th-th uh paint'. Repetitions, e.g. 'don't change, don't change'. Reformulations, e.g. 'it was white so he had to lea- they threw him out'. **Exercise 3** The extracts with the highest informational content are 1 (fable retelling) and 4 (story generation). An explanation involves features of the subjects who are producing these extracts, as well as features of the discourse tasks themselves. In order to retell a fable, a subject must be able to understand and recall the events described in it. Clearly, this is achieved by the subject in Extract 1. Story generation requires the additional ability to draw inferences in order to relate events and characters, and explain characters' motivations for different actions. Once again, the subject in Extract 4 is able to draw these inferences, such as when he infers that the old man and young man must be father and son, and that the young man is leaving home to go to university. The subject in Extract 4 is able to use information in the picture such as the ages of the characters, the presence of books and the sticker on the suitcase to make these inferences. **Exercise 4** The extracts with the lowest informational content are 2 (gist of fables), 3 (lesson of fables), and 5 (proverb meaning). All three discourse tasks require subjects to go beyond the decoding of the semantic meaning of the language used, and draw deeper meanings or truths about life using textual information in combination with world knowledge. In Extract 2, the subject partially achieves this when he identifies the gist of the fable as being about not changing oneself. However, there are so many repetitions and revisions that the amount of information conveyed is outweighed by the amount of language used. A similar scenario occurs in Extract 3, when the subject tries to derive the lesson of the fable. When the subject tries to explain the meaning of the proverb in Extract 5, he runs with a rather literal interpretation of 'swallow' and 'summer' and ends up describing something akin to the migratory pattern of birds at different times of the year. **Exercise 5** (a) True: these subjects are able to attribute thoughts and emotions to the minds of other agents, such as when the subject is able to tell that the old man and dog will miss the young man who is leaving for university.

(b) False: in Extract 5, the subject indicates very clearly that he is aware of his difficulties when he utters 'I'm not doing well with this at all'. (c) False: in Extract 4, the subject is able to recall considerable detail from the picture when it is face down. (d) False: across all extracts, the subjects attend both to the examiner's instructions and to the linguistic stimuli presented to them. (e) False: the subject displays good planning and organization of discourse during story generation. He correctly identifies the key information to be communicated to the examiner, and organizes this information in a logical and coherent way. He begins by setting the temporal context of the story before describing the characters present and their physical and familial relationships to each other. He is also able to describe the emotional states of the characters, a key aspect of good story telling.

6.5   Acquired aphasia 2

Exercise 1 In the months post-stroke, this woman's naming responses move from a pattern where neologistic jargon predominates to a pattern in which she is using semantic jargon (i.e. words that are semantically related to the target word). This transition occurs rapidly following the introduction of a new treatment approach at eight months post-stroke. So it is that at ten months post-onset, the patient's productions of 'scissors', 'flower', 'pencil', 'drinking' and 'cactus' resemble the words 'cut', 'bloom', 'pen', 'cup' and 'prickle', respectively. Her production of 'pencil' could be a phonological error rather than semantic jargon. **Exercise 2** Directions (e.g. south → north); actions (e.g. ride → run); body parts (e.g. knuckles → fingers); temperature (e.g. hot → cold); fruit (e.g. cherry → apple); colour (e.g. green → red); time (e.g. statement of date → statement of time); familial relations (e.g. husband → wife); physical dimensions (e.g. small → big). **Exercise 3** Nouns (e.g. sons → daughters); verbs (e.g. eat → drink); adjectives (e.g. small → big); adverbs (e.g. up → down). JT's substitutions are preserving the grammatical category of the target word. **Exercise 4** (a) hot → cold; (b) knuckles → fingers; (c) husband → wife; (d) cherry → apple. **Exercise 5** (a) Yes: examples are [wɪnər], [hjurər], [kɔkeik] and [radʒ]. (b) Yes: examples are found in (2), (3), (7), (13) and (20). (c) Yes: it seems likely that the use of 'cake' for *triangle* is a visual error. (d) Yes: examples are (15) and (18). (e) Yes: examples are (8) and (9). (f) Yes: an example is the use of 'daughters' and 'children' in (14).

6.5   Acquired aphasia 3

Exercise 1 (a) pentil for 'pencil' (Data 1); trites for 'Sprite' (Data 1); (b) wet for 'cold' (Data 2); hear for 'recognize' (Data 2). **Exercise 2** (a) Request 3 (Data 3); request 5 (Data 3). (b) Request 2 (Data 1); request 6 (Data 2). (c) Request 1 (Data 3); request 2 (Data 3). (d) Request 9 (Data 1); request 4 (Data 2). **Exercise 3** The speaker in Data 3 uses the stereotyped utterance 'Mommy?' **Exercise 4** The questions produced by the speaker in Data 2 are grammatical questions, i.e. they are formed through subject pronoun-auxiliary verb inversion as in 'Do you wanna open this?' The questions produced by the speaker in Data 1 are intonational questions, i.e. they are statements which have a questioning intonation as in 'You open box?' The greater grammatical impairments of this second speaker do not permit him to form grammatical questions. **Exercise 5** Written language, as in request 8 in Data 3 (written word 'German'); body language, as in request 8 in Data 3 (waving of arms); facial expression, as in request 2 in Data 3 (quizzical look).

6.5 Acquired aphasia 4

Exercise 1 The following features of spoken output suggest word-finding problems on the part of these speakers: speakers 1 and 2 make extensive use of unfilled and filled pauses (e.g. uh, um, ur, er, yeah); speaker 1 uses expressions such as 'y'know' and 'sort of' which convey little meaning but allow the speaker to retain his turn; speaker 2 produces an explicit statement 'What's name' which indicates he is struggling to find a target word; speaker 4 uses non-specific vocabulary such as 'stuff' and 'some'. **Exercise 2** Speaker 3 engages in circumlocution when he says 'going to the ground' for *falling*. The following three semantic paraphasias occur: speaker 2 uses 'fee' for *offer*; speaker 3 uses 'bowl' for *sink*; speaker 4 uses 'kitchen' for *sink*. **Exercise 3** The verbal output of speaker 1 displays agrammatism. Nouns (e.g. Kent, blokes, boat) and adjectives (e.g. strange, funny, sudden) are retained in this speaker's verbal output. Articles (definite and indefinite) and pronouns are completely omitted. Prepositions (with the exception of 'of'), conjunctions (with the exception of 'and') and verbs (with the exception of 'waterskiing') are not present. **Exercise 4** Speakers 1 and 2 use non-verbal communication in the form of a mime and hand gesture, respectively. These non-verbal behaviours are serving to compensate for these speakers' word-finding difficulties. **Exercise 5** Speaker 2 displays relatively intact receptive language skills. He readily comprehends the therapist's questions, many of which are syntactically complex and deal with a topic (selling a business) which is complex and not concrete. The cognitive skills of speaker 2 also appear intact. He is clearly aware of, and understands, the negotiations around the selling of his property. He has a clear sense of time (e.g. the time it will take to sell a business). He is able to judge the value of offers he has received. He understands how finance works (e.g. notions like 'capital') and employment and its termination (e.g. redundancy).

6.5 Acquired aphasia 5

Exercise 1 Martha produces a phonemic paraphasic error /breuf/ during her attempted production of 'bread'. **Exercise 2** By describing the function of a phone ('you ring Geraldine on the . . . '), the therapist is providing Martha with a *semantic* cue as an aid to producing the word. **Exercise 3** Speaker AC in Extract 2 is making extensive use of *formulaic* expressions. Three such expressions are (a) 'I came, I saw, I conquered', (b) 'how are you' and (c) 'good morning'. **Exercise 4** Jef uses fillers such as 'euh' and 'ohoh' immediately before a long silence in which he cannot continue what he wants to say. The pronoun 'it' in 'they don't call it out loud' is non-specific suggesting that the speaker is unable to produce a more specific lexeme for what he wants to say. The utterance 'how do I have to say it' reflects some struggle on the speaker's part with finding the words he needs and is also suggestive of a word-finding problem. **Exercise 5** Jef's verbal comprehension skills appear not to be intact. He appears to misunderstand the interviewer's question and returns to talking about the communication skills of the men he has been describing.

6.6 Right-hemisphere language disorder

Exercise 1 There is evidence that P is using humour inappropriately. At the end of P's second turn, he appears to find his remarks funny. However, the examiner's next turn indicates that whatever humour P thinks he has conveyed, it has not been interpreted as such by the examiner. **Exercise 2** P's contribution to the exchange is highly egocentric in nature. The neutral term 'friend' is immediately substituted by the familial term 'son-in-law'. There is extensive reporting of circumstances which are part of P's personal experience (e.g. marital relationships and relationships between a couple and their daughter). **Exercise 3** P's understanding of the metaphor 'is a witch' is concrete and literal in nature. In elaborating the meaning of this metaphor, P refers only to the conventional attributes of witches which are embodied in the semantic meaning of the word 'witch', e.g. inclusion in religious sects, the practice of black magic. **Exercise 4** At one point, it appears that P is aware that his interpretation is not accurate. This is when he denies that having many brooms is part of the meaning of the metaphor: 'My friend's mother-in-law has many brooms . . . no!' However, it seems that this is merely a rejection of one of the conventional attributes of a witch, as he is prepared to accept another conventional attribute, the practice of black magic, as part of the meaning of the metaphor. **Exercise 5** P's use of referring expressions is problematic. In P's second turn in the exchange, he introduces the terms 'she', 'her marriage', and 'her husband', all of which lack clear referents. P is aware of this and immediately establishes a referent by saying 'I'm referring to the mother-in-law of my son-in-law'. But this correction arrives late, and only after the examiner has had to establish a suitable referent for himself.

6.7 Traumatic brain injury

Exercise 1 In the utterance 'Then we found a house and went back home', the listener must draw a number of inferences to connect the finding of the house to the return of the men home. For example, did the owner of the house give the speaker and his brother a set of directions to facilitate their return home? Or did the owner of the house contact the police, who returned the men home? These implicit details must be filled in by the listener in order to comprehend the speaker's narrative. **Exercise 2** The speaker is repetitive in his account of the pig: 'we found a pig in the woods. A pig. Pig got out of my uncle's . . . pig, uh . . . So we found a pig around'. **Exercise 3** (a) There is considerable repetition of Greenfield and Southfield, as well as statements about getting lost. (b) Several abandoned utterances occur, e.g. 'And it doesn't seem . . .'. (c) A subject is omitted in 'I thought ended'. (d) In the utterance 'I got lost there', a referent for 'there' is not established by the speaker. (e) The speaker begins by saying she gets lost going to the hospital. Then, she says she doesn't get lost. Finally, she says again that she does get lost. **Exercise 4** The speaker's use of filled pauses may indicate a word-finding difficulty. Alternatively, these pauses may be indicative of slower information processing speed on the part of the speaker. In both cases, the filled pauses function to retain the speaker's conversational turn while cognitive processing is taking place. **Exercise 5** Notwithstanding their various discourse problems, both speakers are generally successful at establishing cohesive links between utterances. Some examples of these links are: (a) '<u>Me and my brother</u> had been walking into the woods one day and <u>we</u> found a pig . . .' (anaphoric reference). (b) 'I didn't think we were goin' make it back. But we did [make it back]' (verbal ellipsis). (c) 'I don't get lost <u>but</u> I get scared' (conjunction).

6.8 Dementias 1

Exercise 1 The speaker in Extract 1 displays anomia. This is manifested in his inability to produce certain words (e.g. pigeon) and also in the large number of filled pauses (e.g.

Uh, the raven uh-uh, was gonna...). Word-finding difficulties in this subject may be evidence of a memory impairment related to Alzheimer's disease. **Exercise 2** Both extracts fail to address the deeper meanings communicated by the fable in question. In Extract 2, the subject misses the gist of the fable altogether and uses the mention of food to derive a meaning related to the physical survival of animals. In Extract 3, the subject draws an incorrect lesson from the fable about stealing food. **Exercise 3** The subject in Extract 4 is describing a picture rather than generating a story. He describes the characters present (e.g. there is a man), the weather (e.g. it's kind of overcast) and certain actions (e.g. the man and the boy are talking). However, there is no attempt to relate the depicted individuals (e.g. father and son) or describe the deeper significance of the scene, which is the departure of a man's son for university. The subject does not undertake the high-level inferences which are required to obtain these meanings. **Exercise 4** Initially, the subject engages in considerable repetition of the proverb both in whole and in part. Then he produces another proverb – 'There's more than one way to skin a cat' – which he partially succeeds in explaining. But this proverb is unrelated in meaning to the one he has been asked to explain. **Exercise 5** Statement (d).

6.8 Dementias 2

Exercise 1 Subject B.V.: stereotyped utterance (e.g. oh gosh; oh dear); incomplete utterance (e.g. it's um...; Clinton and um...); these utterances reveal that this subject has a word-finding difficulty. **Exercise 2** Subjects RH and EB have problems with topic relevance. Subject RH is at least able to address the examiner's request for his name before veering off onto another topic. Subject EB displays no topic relevance whatsoever. He responds to the examiner's question about the problems he has been having with a response about the tests he has undergone. **Exercise 3** Subject VB is aware of her language problems. This subject describes difficulty with word retrieval. **Exercise 4** Failures of topic relevance suggest problems with pragmatics. The word-finding and word-retrieval difficulties of these subjects also suggest impairment in semantics. **Exercise 5** An assessment of syntax is difficult in these non-fluent PPA subjects because verbal output is largely limited to short phrases and incomplete sentences.

6.8 Dementias 3

Exercise 1 Warren does exhibit problems with the use of syntax. He uses the comparative determiner 'more' without specifying who or what he has more common sense than, e.g. 'I've got more common sense than person X has'. Also, Warren introduces the subordinating conjunction 'if' without including the clause that is necessary to complete the sentence. **Exercise 2** There is no evidence of either a word-finding deficit in Warren's verbal output or an auditory comprehension deficit. **Exercise 3** Initially at least, Warren is able to produce a relevant response to the examiner's questions. However, as soon as he does so, he quickly veers off topic. The large majority of his last utterance is completely irrelevant to the topic of the examiner's question. Topic relevance is an area of considerable impairment for Warren. **Exercise 4** There is evidence of Warren developing meaning associations around the word 'common'. Its first use is in the expression 'common sense' where 'common' has the meaning of the type of thinking and sense employed by each of us. Then Warren presses another meaning of 'common' into use, that of lowly social status. It is this second meaning which becomes the basis of

Warren's extended response to the examiner's question about age. Meaning associations between utterances can also be observed in the spoken output of schizophrenic patients. **Exercise 5** Warren is able to engage in referencing in this exchange. He refers his listener to an earlier part of the conversation in his second utterance (assuming, of course, this is an appropriate use of referencing; he may have said nothing earlier in the conversation about being spoiled). Also, he uses anaphoric reference effectively in his extended utterance at the end. In this way, he introduces his great grandmother into the conversation and then refers to her by the use of 'she'. Also, he introduces a person's name – we are not told what it is – and then refers to this person by the use of 'he'.

Chapter 7: Disorders of voice

Section A: Short-answer questions

7.1 Organic voice disorders

(1) intubation; syndromes; cri du chat; papillomatosis; nodules; abuse; tumour; laryngectomy; artificial/electronic; oesophageal; surgical voice; presbylarynx. **(2)** parts (a), (c) and (d). **(3)** part (c). **(4)** part (a). **(5)** parts (a) and (d). **(6)** part (a). **(7)** parts (a), (c) and (d). **(8)** parts (b) and (d). **(9)** (a) recurrent laryngeal; (b) mucous; glandular; (c) reactive lesion; (d) arytenoid; (e) varices. **(10)** (a) True; (b) False; (c) True; (d) False; (e) False.

7.2 Functional voice disorders

(1) False. **(2)** False. **(3)** True. **(4)** part (c). **(5)** part (b). **(6)** mutation; puberphonia. **(7)** professional; psychological. **(8)** True. **(9)** parts (a), (b) and (c). **(10)** parts (b), (c) and (d).

7.3 Laryngectomy

(1) parts (b) and (d). **(2)** True. **(3)** common; squamous cell; cartilage; radiotherapy; partial; laryngectomy; stoma; respiration; neck; pharynx; voice; prosthesis; trachea; tracheostoma; oesophageal; pitch; restoration; electronic. **(4)** True. **(5)** True. **(6)** False. **(7)** parts (c) and (e). **(8)** parts (a), (b) and (e). **(9)** articulation. **(10)** total.

7.4 Gender dysphoria

(1) part (a). **(2)** False. **(3)** part (d). **(4)** fundamental. **(5)** thyroid cartilage. **(6)** parts (a) and (d). **(7)** parts (a) and (d). **(8)** False. **(9)** True. **(10)** False.

Section B: Data analysis exercises

7.5 Organic voice disorders

Exercise 1 The organic voice disorder characterized in case B is structural in nature. NAR has sulcus vocalis. The factors which are influential in identifying this disorder are: onset of voice problem in childhood, presence of dysphonia in biological relatives, absence of other risk factors (smoking and reflux), spindle-like cleft (unable to achieve full glottal closure), vocal symptoms (suggestive of inadequate glottal closure), treatment (use of fat graft in phonosurgery). **Exercise 2** The organic voice disorder characterized in case A is neurological in nature. NB has adductor spasmodic dysphonia. The factors which are influential in identifying this disorder are: irregular speech breaks (intermittent phonation), vocal symptoms (tense voice, vocal tiredness reflecting intense vocal effort), vocal tremor, absence of structural lesions and oedema, treatment (intramuscular injection of Botulin toxin). **Exercise 3** part (b). **Exercise 4** vocal fold paralysis. **Exercise 5** parts (b) and (d).

7.6   Functional voice disorders

Exercise 1 The functional voice disorder characterized in case B is psychogenic in nature. AB has a psychogenic voice disorder caused by a conversion reaction. The factors which are influential in identifying this disorder are: viral laryngitis followed by dysphonia, no other laryngeal pathology, normal phonation during coughing, able to produce whispered voice, traumatic event (rape) that led to a conflict over speaking out. AB's dysphonia served the purpose of avoiding awareness of emotional conflict and stress which would have been intolerable if directly countenanced. **Exercise 2** The functional voice disorder characterized in case A is hyperfunctional in nature. Judith has muscle tension dysphonia secondary to laryngopharyngeal reflux (LPR). The factors which are influential in identifying this disorder are: primary disorder of LPR indicated by reported symptoms (sensation of fullness in throat and food sticking in throat; frequent coughing) and laryngeal findings (thick mucous strands on folds, oedema, erythema and hypertrophy at back of larynx); secondary disorder of muscle tension dysphonia suggested by vocal abuse behaviours, vocal features (breaks in phonation, low speaking fundamental frequency, breathiness and roughness) and laryngeal findings (medial compression of vocal folds, large posterior glottal chink). **Exercise 3** parts (b), (d) and (e). **Exercise 4** part (c). **Exercise 5** parts (a) and (e).

7.7   Laryngectomy

Exercise 1 Oesophageal voice: Don and Stan. Electronic larynx: Bert and John. Voice prosthesis: Joan and Derek. **Exercise 2** High proficiency: Bert, Don and Joan. Low proficiency: John, Stan and Derek. **Exercise 3** The speaker with a severed tongue nerve is John. **Exercise 4** John is unable to articulate /k/ in 'communication'. The production of this velar plosive requires that the back of the tongue make contact with the velum or soft palate. Because John's tongue nerve has been severed, he is unable to raise the back of his tongue to make contact with the velum. **Exercise 5** wet and gurgly.

7.8   Gender dysphoria

Exercise 1 Subject A achieved a fundamental frequency range between 128 and 155 Hz by the end of therapy. A fundamental frequency of 128 Hz is at the high end of the pitch range for men. Subject B achieved a fundamental frequency of 210 Hz by the end of therapy. This is in the low end of the pitch range for women. **Exercise 2** Subject A, who was a non-smoker, started smoking as a means to achieving a reduction in vocal pitch. Voice therapy will aim to educate the client about safe use of the laryngeal mechanism and will attempt to discourage behaviours like smoking. **Exercise 3** part (a).

Exercise 4 As a MTF transsexual, subject B is likely to receive hormone therapy consisting of oestrogens, progesterone and testosterone-blocking agents. There is evidence that oestrogen therapy produces only minor changes in pitch. The relative insensitivity of the larynx to oestrogen therapy explains why subject B's hormone therapy appears to hold less significance than subject A's androgen therapy during the respective attempts of these clients to achieve pitch alterations. **Exercise 5** Subject B is receiving visual feedback on the pitch of her voice through the use of a Visi-pitch display.

Chapter 8: Disorders of fluency

Section A: Short-answer questions

8.1   Developmental stuttering

(**1**) genetic; 2:1; 4:1; three; resolve; iterations; perseverations; syllable; phoneme; vowel; duration; pet starter; schwa; circumlocution; covert; interiorized; secondaries; dysfluency. (**2**) part (a). (**3**) part (d). (**4**) True. (**5**) False. (**6**) parts (a) and (c). (**7**) parts (a), (b) and (d). (**8**) True. (**9**) parts (a), (b) and (c). (**10**) parts (b), (c) and (e).

8.2   Acquired stuttering

(**1**) True. (**2**) True. (**3**) False. (**4**) part (c). (**5**) parts (c) and (d). (**6**) dysarthria; stroke; neurological; aphasia; lesion; subcortical; psychological. (**7**) parts (c) and (e). (**8**) True. (**9**) True. (**10**) False.

8.3   Cluttering

(**1**) parts (c), (d) and (e). (**2**) True. (**3**) True. (**4**) False. (**5**) parts (a) and (c). (**6**) parts (a) and (b). (**7**) False. (**8**) True. (**9**) rate. (**10**) epidemiology.

Section B: Data analysis exercises

8.4   Developmental stuttering

Exercise 1 Plosives (e.g. /t/) and fricatives (e.g. /s/) are the two classes of sounds most often involved in word-initial repetitions. **Exercise 2** During the production of 'the World Cup', there is evidence of the use of a creaky voice, as indicated by the symbol V̰ from the Voice Quality Symbols system. **Exercise 3** NS uses the velopharyngeal fricative [fŋ] during repetitions in the production of 'the top nations' and 'provincial towns'. Children who have a cleft palate can also use this sound during speech production. The symbol for the velopharyngeal fricative is part of the extended International Phonetic Alphabet. **Exercise 4** During repetitions in NS's speech, there are fluctuations in loudness. For example, during the production of 'the top nations', NS uses quiet speech initially (indicated by *p* in curly brackets) and then uses loud speech (indicated by *f* in curly brackets). During production of 'provincial towns', NS uses quiet speech at the start of his repetition which becomes quieter speech (indicated by *pp*) as the repetition continues. These symbols for degrees of loudness are from the Voice Quality

Symbols system. **Exercise 5** Ejective consonants are used by NS including the alveolar ejective [t'] and alveolar fricative ejective [s']. A pulmonic ingressive airstream mechanism is used during the production of 'towns' and 'semi-finals'. Alongside fluctuations in loudness, these airstream anomalies indicate that NS has significant difficulties with breath support for speech.

8.5   Acquired stuttering 1

Exercise 1 Whole-word and part-word repetitions are common in SS's speech. Whole-word repetition occurs only on words of one syllable (e.g. 'we', 'got'), a pattern that is similar to the whole-word repetitions observed in relation to developmental stuttering. Part-word repetitions involve CV or CCV syllables (e.g. [mə] and [kreɪ]). The vowel which is repeated in these syllables is the vowel of the target word. However, in developmental stuttering a schwa vowel is most likely to be repeated and then replaced by the vowel of the target word. In only one instance in the data did SS repeat and then replace the schwa vowel (see 'with'). **Exercise 2** Sound prolongations or perseverations are not evident in SS's speech. These sound errors are found in developmental stuttering. **Exercise 3** This does not occur in words of more than one syllable which are produced by SS. These words are uttered as discrete syllables rather than a fluent whole (see how SS produces 'supplies', 'navy' and 'Monday', for example). In SS's case, part-word repetitions only lead to the fluent production of the whole target word when that word is a monosyllable. **Exercise 4** In the production of 'apartment', SS appears to inch forward in the word by attempting each syllable sequence. **Exercise 5** In only one of these repetitions – the word 'parachute' – is the target word produced during the repetition sequence. In all the other repetitions, units short of the target word are produced during the repetition sequence.

8.5   Acquired stuttering 2

Exercise 1 Choose from among the following possibilities: (a) A displays syllable and word repetitions which are not seen in developmental stuttering. (b) A exhibits none of the secondary behaviours which are often (but not always) found in developmental stuttering. (c) A's stuttering did not cease during choral reading. Choral reading and a number of other conditions are known to induce immediate fluency in individuals with developmental stuttering. (d) A exhibited an increased pitch of voice. This is not seen in developmental stuttering. (e) A did not use starters. Starters are often (but not always) seen in developmental stuttering. (f) A did not display specific word fears, which is often seen in developmental stuttering. (g) A did not display situational fears (e.g. speaking in public), which is often seen in developmental stuttering. **Exercise 2** part (b).
Exercise 3 The following features of A's case made a conversion reaction a plausible explanation of his stuttering behaviour: (a) Stuttering had an acute onset. (b) The onset of stuttering was contemporaneous with a period of stress in A's life. (c) There were no motor or other neurological signs (with the exception of the problem with writing). (d) All initial neurological examinations (e.g. MRI) were normal. (e) A's elevated pitch appeared to be explained by the increased tension in the area of his shoulders and neck. **Exercise 4** parts (a) and (c). **Exercise 5** part (e).

8.6   Cluttering

Exercise 1 Two features of motoric cluttering are: (a) fast phoneme repetitions (e.g. t t t today), and (b) short pauses at inappropriate junctures. **Exercise 2** Two features of linguistic cluttering are: language is generally disorganized and confused as evidenced by (a) a preponderance of fillers (e.g. well, er, um), and (b) excessive phrase and sentence revision (e.g. the heat, well, the er, the er, climate really . . .). **Exercise 3** The phoneme repetitions produced by speaker A are similar to the iterations of single sounds in word- and syllable-initial position which are observed in stuttering. **Exercise 4** Word-finding difficulty. **Exercise 5** The pauses used by speaker A split subjects from their verbs (e.g. I (:) took the bus) and articles from their nouns (e.g. a (:) service). Pauses in normal speech observe grammatical boundaries.

Chapter 9: Hearing disorders

Section A: Short-answer questions

9.1   Conductive hearing loss

(1) (a) conductive; (b) sensorineural; (c) sensorineural; (d) conductive; (e) conductive. **(2)** middle ear; Eustachian tube; cleft palate; tensor veli palatini; ventilation; ossicles; malleus; stapes; smallest; suppurative; tympanic membrane; external auditory meatus; perforations; myringotomy; pressure-equalizing; middle ear. **(3)** parts (a), (b) and (e). **(4)** part (b). **(5)** parts (d) and (e). **(6)** tympanometry. **(7)** conductive hearing loss. **(8)** (a) False; (b) True; (c) False; (d) True; (e) True. **(9)** parts (d) and (e). **(10)** parts (a), (c) and (d).

9.2   Sensorineural hearing loss

(1) parts (a), (c) and (e). **(2)** parts (a), (d) and (e). **(3)** hearing loss; normal; tinnitus; intolerance; directional; cochlear; basilar; stereocilia; cell body; threshold shift; presbycusis. **(4)** parts (a) and (b). **(5)** parts (b), (d) and (e). **(6)** acoustic nerve tumour. **(7)** auditory cortical centres. **(8)** sensorineural hearing loss. **(9)** parts (a), (c) and (e). **(10)** (a) False; (b) False; (c) True; (d) False; (e) True.

9.3   Cochlear implantation

(1) False. **(2)** part (a). **(3)** parts (a), (b) and (c). **(4)** False. **(5)** True. **(6)** parts (a), (b), (d) and (e). **(7)** cochlea; disabilities; educational; quicker; postlingually; congenital; critical period; intellectual; meningitis; oral; total; auditory. **(8)** True. **(9)** parts (a), (b) and (d). **(10)** central.

Section B: Data analysis exercises

9.4   Congenital hearing loss 1

Exercise 1 (a) cream [tərim]; swim [dəwɪm]. (b) Choose from: mean to [min ə stu]; it [ɪçt]; new dog [nusdɔχk]; tell [tsɛ]. (c) roof [βupf]; piece [pitsi]. (d) Choose from: wish [fwɪt]; we [ɸwi]; read [vrid]. (e) Choose from: name [ndæ] [neɪmp]; my [mbaɪ]; man [mbænt]. **Exercise 2** moving [mufvĩ]. **Exercise 3** toothpaste [tuθpeɪs]; everybody [æfrtpɑdi]. **Exercise 4** ball [bwa]; paste [breɪs]. **Exercise 5** There is mistiming of velar movement. The velum is lowering at the point where it needs to close to produce /p/.

9.4   Congenital hearing loss 2

Exercise 1 Ear canal stenosis and atresia, and ossicular defects are responsible for conductive hearing loss in BOR syndrome. In Stickler syndrome, a quite different pathology is the basis of conductive hearing loss. In this case, conductive hearing loss is related to recurrent otitis media with effusion. **Exercise 2** In BOR syndrome, sensorineural hearing loss is related to cochlear hypoplasia. Although the causal mechanism for sensorineural hearing loss in Stickler syndrome is less clear, inner ear structures are likely to be compromised by the collagen abnormality in the disorder and by alterations in the pigmented epithelium of the inner ear. **Exercise 3** Progressive hearing loss in BOR syndrome is believed to be related to the enlargement of the vestibular aqueduct. **Exercise 4** Both syndromes display pathological features which are normally contraindications for cochlear implants. The lack of cochlear development (cochlear hypoplasia) in BOR syndrome and recurrent otitis media with effusion in Stickler syndrome are the pathological features in question. **Exercise 5** Only in Stickler syndrome is speech likely to be hypernasal in nature. Hypernasality in this syndrome is related to velopharyngeal incompetence, which is a consequence of the palatal defects (cleft palate) that are a commonly observed feature of the syndrome.

9.4   Congenital hearing loss 3

Exercise 1 parts (a), (c) and (e). **Exercise 2** Microtia and atresia frequently occur together because the outer ear and middle ear develop from a common embryological origin. **Exercise 3** George has a conductive hearing loss which is related to atresia of the ear canal. However, there may also be a sensorineural component to his hearing loss which is related to the temporal cortical atrophy revealed by a CT scan. **Exercise 4** The same palatal defect which causes velopharyngeal insufficiency is also responsible for impaired opening of the Eustachian tube and a consequent lack of middle ear ventilation. In the absence of adequate ventilation, the middle ear is at risk of otitis media with effusion, which is a further cause of conductive hearing loss. It emerges that George's conductive hearing loss is likely to have two significant, but different, causal pathologies – ear canal atresia and otitis media with effusion. **Exercise 5** parts (b) and (d).

9.4   Congenital hearing loss 4

Exercise 1 The palatal muscles which control the opening and closing of the velopharyngeal port also control the function of the Eustachian tube which connects the nasopharynx to the middle ear. These muscles are clearly impaired to some degree in NC on account of the cleft of her soft palate. The failure of these muscles to function normally will lead to velopharyngeal insufficiency and associated speech hypernasality on the one hand, and inadequate ventilation of the middle ear with consequent otitis media and conductive hearing loss on the other hand. **Exercise 2** It is clearly not possible to map hearing loss directly onto the vowel and consonant inventories of children – many other factors which are unrelated to hearing, for example, speech motor skills, also play a significant role in the sounds that a child can and cannot produce. With this proviso in place, it is possible to say that NC's hearing loss of 30 dB HL (a mild hearing loss) largely spares her perception of vowel sounds, while rendering her perception of certain consonant sounds (e.g. voiceless consonants) impossible. To the extent that the sounds which NC can perceive are the ones she goes on to produce, NC's vowel production will be superior to her production of consonants. **Exercise 3** We are told that NC's hearing loss of 30 dB HL is more severe in the low frequencies. /z/ and /v/ are low frequency sounds and are unlikely to be perceived and therefore produced by NC. However, /f/ is a high frequency sound and, as such, may be somewhat more easily perceived and then produced by NC. **Exercise 4** There is a visual dimension to the articulation of /f/ – this consonant has a labiodental place of articulation – which is lacking in the case of alveolar /s/. The child with hearing loss is sensitive to this visual dimension of the articulation of speech sounds even as he or she is unable to perceive them auditorily. This visual information may then be used to develop a motor program for the production of the sound. This same explanation may account for the superior production of /v/ over /z/ and /m/ over /n/. The former sound in each case has a visual dimension to the articulation (labiodental and bilabial places of articulation, respectively) which is lacking in the case of alveolar sounds. **Exercise 5** NC also has a tongue ankylosis which may further contribute to her difficulty in producing alveolar sounds.

9.5 Sensorineural hearing loss 1

Exercise 1 (a) skate [kejt]; star [ta]. (b) keys [ti]; dad [da]. (c) shoe [tu]; pencil [pɛn̪t̪ə]. (d) radio [weio]; blocks [bwɔt̪ʂ]. **Exercise 2** (a) carrots [teə]. (b) car [ka]. **Exercise 3** Stopping occurs in word-initial (e.g. shoe [tu]), word-medial (e.g. pencil [pɛn̪t̪ə]) and word-final (e.g. house [hawt̪]) positions. **Exercise 4** Nasal assimilation. **Exercise 5** scissor [ɟit̪ə]; pencil [pɛn̪t̪ə].

9.5 Sensorineural hearing loss 2

Exercise 1 parts (a), (b), (d) and (e). **Exercise 2** All three children exhibit middle ear pathology. The boy in Case A has an abnormal left ear tympanogram, and required a myringotomy and insertion of a pressure equalizing tube. The child in Case B displayed significant negative pressure on acoustic impedance measurements in both ears, and was recommended medication to treat a middle ear problem by his otolaryngologist. The child in Case C also had negative pressure in his right ear during acoustic impedance testing. **Exercise 3** part (c). **Exercise 4** The boy in Case B is likely to have otitis media with effusion (OME). This is suggested by the significant negative pressure found in both ears during acoustic impedance measurements. When this study was conducted in 1981, the standard treatment for OME involved some combination of decongestants, antihistamines, steroids and antibiotics. However, recent clinical guidance recommends that none of these medications should be used in the treatment of OME. It is difficult to say with certainty if the recommended treatment was successful, because although a normal tympanogram was obtained for the left ear following treatment, significant negative pressure remained in the right ear. It is always possible that the left ear improvement may well have occurred in the absence of medication. **Exercise 5** The first three formants are the most important for the correct recognition of English vowels. The frequency response of the first, second and third formants is 250–1000 Hz, 1000–2000 Hz, and 2000–3000 Hz, respectively. Given this child's improvement in his hearing in the right ear at 500–2000 Hz, it is likely that his perception of vowel sounds will be relatively spared. However, this child's significant decrement in hearing at 4000 and 8000 Hz will adversely affect his perception of certain consonant sounds. For example, the fricative consonants /z, s/ have energy in the frequency region of 3500 through 8000 Hz, and are less likely to be perceived correctly by this child.

9.6   Cochlear implantation 1

Exercise 1 (a) feet – fat. (b) fell – shell. (c) bat – pat. (d) bat – mat. (e) beet – boot. **Exercise 2** (a) van – fan: voiced labiodental vs. voiceless labiodental; two – shoe: stop vs. fricative; pea – key: bilabial vs. velar place of articulation; boot – boat: high vs. mid vowel height; goat – coat: voiced velar vs. voiceless velar; pie – tie: bilabial vs. alveolar place of articulation. (b) bear – pear (one: voicing); pat – fat (two: manner of articulation; place of articulation); pea – paw (two: vowel height and vowel backness); pat – cat (one: place of articulation); two – shoe (two: manner of articulation; place of articulation). **Exercise 3** This finding indicates that the relationship between the perception and production of sound contrasts in minimal pairs in children with cochlear implants is rather tenuous and that these skills may need to be addressed separately in remediation. **Exercise 4** These correlations reveal that stress and resonance quality are directly related to the amount of auditory experience accrued by children with cochlear implants. Although these prosodic and voice variables were still markedly impaired in these children – as they are in hearing impaired children without cochlear implants – there is still the possibility of their improvement given the auditory experience that is made possible by early implantation. **Exercise 5** The term 'nasopharyngeal' describes a type of 'backed' (pharyngeal) resonance rather than forward (oral) resonance. It includes classic cul-de-sac resonance that is often associated with the speech of individuals with hearing impairment.

9.6   Cochlear implantation 2

Exercise 1 This finding suggests that the level of auditory stimulation provided by this child's hearing aid was unlikely to be adequate for the development of the central auditory pathways. **Exercise 2** The lesion which affects hearing in the left ear may be extensive and may involve the acoustic nerve or central auditory pathway. Certainly, this is suggested by the fact that there was no response to sound at any frequency in the left ear. A lesion of this type is a contraindication for a cochlear implant which can only function if the acoustic nerve and central auditory pathway are intact. **Exercise 3** An implant is contraindicated for the right ear, as this child has microtia and atresia of this ear. Atresia, particularly when complete, is associated with severe conductive hearing loss. **Exercise 4** Simple behavioural observation of auditory behaviour in children can be misleading, and can lead to misdiagnosis and mismanagement of the hearing-impaired child. For this reason, a cross-check principle has been advocated in paediatric audiometry. This principle recommends the use of physiological test procedures, such as auditory brainstem response, as cross-checks of behavioural test results. **Exercise 5** The child in Case A was a full 12 months younger than the child in Case B when cochlear implantation was conducted (19 months of age versus 2;7 years). The poorer outcome of the child in Case B suggests that a vital period of time for the auditory stimulation of the central auditory pathways has been missed, but successfully harnessed by cochlear implantation for the child in Case A. The limited compliance of the child in Case B – he did not wear his implant consistently – has also probably contributed to his poorer outcome.

Glossary

accessory feature: also known as secondary behaviours; describes an extensive range of verbal and non-verbal behaviours which occur alongside stuttering (e.g. eye blinking).

acoustic neuroma: a benign tumour that is also known as vestibular schwannoma. Acoustic neuroma is the most commonly occurring tumour in the head and neck. When of sufficient size, it can appear on a CAT or MRI scan, but is often detectable before then using an auditory brainstem response test. Symptoms include hearing loss, tinnitus and imbalance.

acoustic reflex test: a test which is based on the signal threshold level at which the stapedial muscle contracts. The lowest signal intensity which is capable of eliciting this acoustic reflex is known as the acoustic reflex threshold. The acoustic reflex test is a sensitive indicator of cochlear pathology.

aetiology: the medical or other causes of a disorder. Causes may range from organic problems (e.g. a laryngeal tumour in a voice disorder) through to psychological and behavioural factors (e.g. the communication impairment in selective mutism). Many communication disorders have a mixed aetiology, with organic, psychological and behavioural factors all contributing to the development of these disorders.

agnosia: a condition in which an affected individual is unable to recognize visual stimuli (visual agnosia) or auditory stimuli (auditory agnosia) despite having no sensory impairment (e.g. a patient will have a normal audiogram). If the recognition of spoken words is compromised, a verbal auditory agnosia is diagnosed. If the recognition of environmental sounds is disrupted, a nonverbal auditory agnosia is diagnosed. Verbal auditory agnosia is one of the first presenting signs of Landau-Kleffner syndrome.

agrammatism: a feature of non-fluent aphasia (hence, the term 'agrammatic' aphasia) in which the speaker retains content words but omits function words and inflectional morphemes from his or her speech; verbal output has the appearance of a telegram, e.g. 'Man . . . walk . . . dog' for *The man is walking the dog.*

AIDS dementia complex: also referred to as AIDS-related dementia, AIDS encephalopathy and HIV encephalopathy. The condition is characterized by a progressive deterioration in cognitive function, including language, which is accompanied by motor abnormalities and behavioural changes. The association of cognitive changes with motor and behavioural signs is denoted by the word 'complex'.

Alzheimer's disease (AD): a neurodegenerative disease that is the most frequent cause of dementia; amyloid plaques and neurofibrillary tangles develop in the brains of AD sufferers.

amyotrophic lateral sclerosis: *see* **motor neurone disease**

anomia: the inability of an adult with aphasia to access the spoken names of objects and concepts despite having the articulatory skills to produce these names if they could be retrieved. If this inability occurs alongside normal comprehension and fluent sentence production, then the patient is described as having anomic aphasia.

Apert's syndrome: a genetic disorder which is caused by mutations in the FGFR2 gene; features include premature fusion of certain skull bones (craniosynostosis), fusion of fingers and toes (syndactyly), conductive hearing loss, and cognitive abilities which can range from normal to mild or moderate intellectual disability.

aphasia (dysphasia): an acquired language disorder in which the expression and/or reception of language (spoken, written and signed) is compromised. Aphasia can be broadly classified as fluent and non-fluent types. Fluent aphasia is further subdivided into Wernicke's, anomic, conduction and transcortical sensory aphasia. Non-fluent aphasia is further subdivided into Broca's and transcortical motor aphasia. A further non-fluent aphasia – global aphasia – is characterized by severe impairment of all language functions.

apraxia (dyspraxia): a motor disorder which can affect speech production (verbal dyspraxia), the movement of limbs (limb dyspraxia), the movement of oral structures (oral dyspraxia), etc.; the dominant terms to describe the speech disorder in children and adults are childhood apraxia of speech and apraxia of speech, respectively.

articulatory groping: the deliberate, conscious placement of the articulators to achieve speech sound production; a feature of developmental verbal dyspraxia and apraxia of speech.

artificial larynx: also known as an electronic larynx, this hand-held device is positioned against the neck by the laryngectomee from where it vibrates air in the oral cavity to produce voice; can be used on its own as the sole method of communication or in combination with other forms of non-laryngeal voice production.

atrophy: the wasting or loss of muscle tissue either through lack of use (disuse atrophy) or damage of a nerve that innervates a muscle (neurogenic atrophy). Vocal fold atrophy can occur in the client with vocal fold paralysis.

attention deficit hyperactivity disorder (ADHD): a disorder that is diagnosed on the basis of symptoms of inattention and hyperactivity-impulsivity; there are three main subtypes of ADHD: a combined type; a predominantly inattentive type; a predominantly hyperactive-impulsive type.

audiology: the study of hearing; also, the profession which is concerned with the prevention, diagnosis and rehabilitation of auditory problems.

auditory brainstem response: this technique is an evoked potentials measurement of the auditory nervous system. Through electrodes taped to the skull, signals are delivered to each ear independently. Microvolt sensory responses from the auditory nerve and brainstem are detected through these electrodes. Slight modifications of the auditory brainstem response technique permit measurement of the middle latency response, an evoked response that occurs between the brainstem and auditory cortex.

augmentative and alternative communication (AAC): when spoken communication skills are severely impaired and are unlikely to improve, a type of AAC may be considered for use with a client. AAC may take high- and low-tech forms such as a communication board attached to a client's wheelchair or the use of synthesized speech output.

aural atresia: a congenital condition in which the ear canal fails to develop normally. Aural atresia is associated with many craniofacial syndromes including Treacher Collins syndrome and Crouzon's syndrome. It is often accompanied by middle ear deformities.

autism spectrum disorder: a neurodevelopmental disorder in which there are persistent deficits in social communication and social interaction across multiple contexts and restricted, repetitive patterns of behaviour, interests, or activities. Symptoms must be present in the early developmental period and must cause clinically significant impairment in social, occupational, or other important areas of functioning.

benign rolandic epilepsy: also known as benign childhood epilepsy with centrotemporal spikes. Benign rolandic epilepsy is the most common idiopathic focal epilepsy in children. The condition is described as 'benign' because of the absence of neurological deficits, infrequent focal somatosensory or motor seizures which occur predominantly during sleep, reasonable response to medication and spontaneous resolution before 15 to 16 years of age.

bipolar disorder: formerly known as manic depression, this is a psychiatric disorder in which the patient's mood alters between manic episodes (characterized by euphoria, restlessness, poor judgement and risk-taking behaviour), depressive episodes (characterized by depression, anxiety and hopelessness), and episodes of normal mood (known as euthymia).

birth anoxia: a lack of oxygen during the birth process. Anoxia can cause cerebral damage in conditions such as cerebral palsy.

bradykinesia: slowness of movement. Bradykinesia is one of the cardinal manifestations of Parkinson's disease.

branchio-oto-renal (BOR) syndrome: an autosomal dominant disorder in which there is abnormal development of the first and second branchial arches. The disorder has a phenotype consisting of branchial, otological and renal defects.

central auditory processing disorder (CAPD): also known as auditory processing disorder. Damage to any part of the central auditory nervous system, from the cochlear nucleus in the brainstem to the auditory cortex, may result in CAPD. Specifically, CAPD is not related to higher-order language or cognitive factors. A range of auditory skills and abilities are compromised in CAPD including sound localization and lateralization, auditory discrimination, auditory pattern recognition, temporal aspects of audition, and auditory performance in competing or degraded acoustic signals.

cerebral palsy: a neurodevelopmental disorder that results in impairment of gross and fine motor skills, speech production included; cerebral palsy is caused by a range of factors in the pre-, peri- and postnatal periods which cause damage to the brain's motor centres.

cerebrovascular accident (CVA): the medical term for a stroke; CVAs may be caused by a blood clot (embolus) in one of the blood vessels in the brain or leading to the brain (embolic stroke) or by a haemorrhage (haemorrhagic stroke) in one of these vessels.

cholesteatoma: a middle ear disorder in which a benign accumulation of epithelium grows superiorly in the attic of the tympanic membrane. As it grows, cholesteatoma may erode away the ossicles.

circumlocution: means literally to talk ('locution') around ('circum') a word; circumlocutions are used by aphasic speakers when they cannot retrieve a target word and stutterers who are trying to avoid words that will cause them to block.

cleft lip and palate: a disorder of embryological development that results in a cleft of the upper lip, alveolus, hard and soft palates; clefts may be unilateral or bilateral and can affect the primary palate only, the secondary palate only or both primary and secondary palates. Some clefts of the palate are described as submucous in nature, because the mucous membrane covering the palate may be intact and conceal an absence of muscle and bone beneath it.

cluttering: a fluency disorder which is characterized by increased rate of speech, disorganized language and (somewhat disputed) a lack of awareness of communication difficulties on the part of the speaker; most often found alongside stuttering but sometimes occurs in a pure form.

cochlear aplasia: a congenital malformation of the inner ear in which there is no cochlea and normal or malformed vestibule and semicircular canals.

cochlear implant: a surgically implanted electronic device which is coupled to external components and provides useful hearing to children and adults with severe-to-profound sensorineural hearing loss.

cognitive-communication disorder: the term applied to any communication disorder which is related to cognitive deficits. The language and communication impairments of clients with traumatic brain injury and right-hemisphere damage are described as cognitive-communication disorders.

computerized axial tomography (CAT): a technique in which an X-ray source produces a narrow, fan-shaped beam of X-rays to irradiate a section of the body. On a single rotation of the X-ray source around the body, many different 'snapshots' are taken. These are then reconstructed by a computer into a cross-sectional image of internal organs and tissues for each complete rotation.

conduct disorder: a disorder in which an individual displays a persistent and repetitive pattern of behaviour that violates the basic rights of others or age-appropriate societal norms or rules. Behaviours include aggression to people and animals and destruction of property. The behaviour disturbance causes clinically significant impairment in social, academic or occupational functioning.

conductive hearing loss: a hearing loss which is related to damage and disease of the outer and middle ear, leading to compromised conduction of sound waves; causes include the failure of the ear canal to develop during embryological development (resulting in complete atresia of the ear canal), the development of middle ear disease such as otitis media ('glue ear') and ossification of the ossicular chain in otosclerosis.

contact ulcer: *see* **granuloma**

conversion aphonia: loss of voice, most commonly in females, in response to a traumatic event or some other psychological stressor; vocal folds can still adduct sufficiently to perform vegetative functions (e.g. coughing) but not for the purpose of voicing.

covert stuttering: also known as interiorized stuttering. Covert stuttering occurs when the person who stutters becomes so adept at hiding their stuttering that the casual listener (or even speech-language pathologists) may not detect overt signs of stuttering in the person's speech. The person with a covert stutter has typically developed an extensive range of avoidance strategies to maintain the appearance of normal fluency.

craniofacial syndrome: any syndrome in which there are congenital malformations of the bones of the face and skull (cranium). These syndromes have implications for speech and hearing on account of their disruption of the anatomical structures which are integral to both processes. Significant examples for speech-language pathologists are Apert's syndrome, Crouzon's syndrome and Treacher Collins syndrome.

Creutzfeldt-Jakob disease: a neurodegenerative disease characterized by spongiform change in the brain, neuronal loss and proliferation of astrocytes (specialized glial cells that contiguously line the entire central nervous system). The disease has sporadic, familial and iatrogenic forms and, more recently, a variant form which is related to BSE in cattle. Affected individuals develop dementia.

cricothyroid approximation: a surgical procedure undertaken in transsexual clients to achieve elevation of the pitch of the voice; titanium sutures are used to draw the cricoid and thyroid cartilages of the larynx together, thus stretching the vocal folds.

cri du chat syndrome: a rare genetic disorder which is associated with a partial deletion on the short arm of chromosome 5. The disorder is characterized by a high-pitched cry in infancy and childhood, from which the syndrome derives its name (literally, 'cry of the cat'). Children with this syndrome present with physical and cognitive problems, including malocclusion, hyper- and hypotonia, delayed motor development, microcephaly, mild-to-profound intellectual disability, a short attention span, and a range of problematic behaviours (e.g. hyperactivity, aggression).

crossed aphasia: aphasia following a right-hemisphere lesion in right-handed individuals. Cases of crossed aphasia are relatively uncommon.

cytomegalovirus (CMV): the most common cause of congenital infection in the US. Congenital CMV infection is the leading cause of sensorineural hearing loss in young children and can also cause significant intellectual disability. CMV is also a common opportunistic infection in individuals with HIV infection.

dementia: a deterioration in higher cortical functions (e.g. language, memory) that can be caused by a range of diseases (e.g. vascular disease, Alzheimer's disease), infections (e.g. HIV infection) and lifestyle (e.g. alcohol-related dementia).

derailment: a feature of formal thought disorder in schizophrenia, in which utterances slip or shift from one topic to another without bridging concepts.

developmental phonological disorder: a condition in which children misarticulate many more speech sounds than is expected for their age. The disorder occurs in the absence of factors such as neuromuscular impairment and intellectual disability which might otherwise explain speech sound errors. Errors are typically characterized in terms of phonological processes such as stopping, fronting and weak syllable deletion. The disorder is more commonly found in boys than in girls.

diadochokinesis (DDK): rapid syllable repetitions, e.g. /pə, tə, kə/, can be used to examine alternating articulatory movements and are a test of oral diadochokinesis; DDK rates are a routine part of the assessment of many speech disorders, e.g. apraxia of speech.

Down's syndrome: a chromosomal disorder that results from an extra chromosome 21; this additional chromosome may be found in all cells (trisomy 21), in some cells (mosaic) or attached to another chromosome (translocation); Down's syndrome results in physical problems (e.g. heart defects) and cognitive difficulties (intellectual disability).

dysarthria: a speech disorder that is caused by damage to the central and peripheral nervous systems; can be developmental or acquired in nature and affects articulation, resonation, respiration, phonation and prosody.

dysfluency: any disruption in the flow of speech. The term is used most commonly of the iterations and perseverations of stuttered speech, but dysfluency is also a feature of other communication disorders (e.g. aphasia).

dysgraphia: the name of a disorder of written language that is typically found in adults as part of an aphasia; the disorder is linguistic in nature rather than the result of motor difficulties which preclude the use of a pen to form letters.

dyslexia: a reading impairment which can be found in children (developmental dyslexia) and in adults (acquired dyslexia). There are different types of dyslexia. For example, the individual with deep dyslexia can read words with concrete meanings more easily than words with abstract meanings. In surface dyslexia, which is often found in semantic dementia, the reading of non-words is preserved while the reading of irregular words is impaired.

dysphagia: the term given to a swallowing disorder in children and adults. Dysphagia can arise following a stroke (neurogenic dysphagia), as a result of structural causes (e.g. a tumour), as a complication of surgery (iatrogenic dysphagia) or on account of psychological factors (psychogenic dysphagia). In most cases, the disorder can be managed by dietary and other modifications. When dysphagia is severe, non-oral feeding is instituted as the only safe method of feeding.

dysphonia: another term for a voice disorder. Dysphonias may be organic (i.e. have a structural or neurological aetiology) or functional in nature (i.e. have a psychogenic or hyperfunctional aetiology). Regardless of the origin of a dysphonia, its effect on the perceptual attributes of the voice may be captured by terms such as 'hoarse', 'breathy' and 'strain-strangled'.

dysthymia: a chronic type of depression in which a person's moods are regularly low, but symptoms are not as severe as those found in major depression.

echolalia: the repetition of another speaker's utterance either immediately (immediate echolalia) or after several conversational turns (delayed echolalia); found in individuals with autism and in some speakers with aphasia.

electroencephalography (EEG): a non-invasive technique in which the brain's electrical activity is recorded by means of electrodes placed on the scalp. Given that this electrical activity is small – it is measured in microvolts – the signal must be amplified before a resultant trace can be made. Although EEG has good temporal resolution (brain activity can be recorded almost as soon as it happens), the technique cannot locate the source of a signal. Functional MRI (fMRI) has better spatial resolution than EEG.

electroglottography (EGG): a non-invasive technique that indexes the contact area between the vocal folds. Two electrodes are secured around the neck at the level of the larynx. The opening and closing of the folds causes variation in the electrical resistance of a small, high-frequency current which is passed between the electrodes. These changes in resistance are displayed onscreen. Electroglottography can be used to assess and treat voice disorders, the latter through the provision of visual feedback.

electromyography (EMG): a technique which is used to record electrical activity in muscle. Recordings are made using a disposable concentric needle electrode which is inserted into the muscle. The technique has a range of clinical applications. For example, it can be used to demonstrate widespread denervation and fasciculation in motor neurone disease, thus confirming the diagnosis of the disorder.

electropalatography (EPG): an instrumental technique that provides a visual display of tongue-palate contacts; used in the assessment and treatment of a range of individuals including children with cleft palate, although not all subjects can tolerate the artificial palate that must be worn in this technique.

emotional and behavioural disorder: a disorder in which affected individuals commonly engage in behaviours (e.g. verbal and physical aggression) that negatively influence their ability to negotiate peer and adult relationships and their educational experience.

epidemiology: the study of the prevalence and incidence of a disease or disorder. Prevalence describes the total number of cases of a disease or disorder which exist in a population. Incidence captures the number of newly diagnosed cases of a disease or disorder, typically within a year.

executive dysfunction: executive functions are a group of cognitive skills which are essential to goal-directed behaviour (e.g. planning ability, mental flexibility) and which are believed to be mediated in large part by the brain's frontal lobes; impairment of these cognitive skills is thought to be related to communication difficulties in clients who sustain a traumatic brain injury, among others.

fasciculation: fine, rapid, flickering and sometimes worm-like twitching of a portion of muscle. In the tongue, fasciculations may be observed as small movements on the tongue surface. Fasciculations can be observed in healthy persons and in clients with neurological disorders (e.g. motor neurone disease).

fat graft: injection of autologous fat into the vocal folds as a means of augmenting soft tissue defects (e.g. sulcus vocalis) and other laryngeal anomalies. Fat grafts can be used to treat unilateral vocal fold paralysis, where the extra bulk created by the graft eliminates glottic air leak and breathy dysphonia.

festination: originally described as a disturbance of gait in patients with Parkinson's disease. Such clients have difficulty initiating locomotion. However, when they start walking, they rapidly accelerate to the point where they are unable to stop. Festination is also observed in the handwriting and speech of clients with Parkinson's disease.

FG syndrome: an X-linked recessive disorder which is predominantly found in males. The disorder is characterized by physical and cognitive abnormalities including cardiac defects, short stature, intellectual disability and unusual facial features (e.g. prominent forehead).

flight of ideas: a feature of manic discourse in which topical shifts are accompanied by pressured speech (excessive speech produced at a rapid rate) and may include wordplay; rarely found in schizophrenia.

foetal alcohol syndrome: a set of birth defects caused by pre-natal exposure of the foetus to alcohol; characteristics include abnormal facial features, growth deficiencies and central nervous system defects (e.g. intellectual disability); the phenotypic expression of this syndrome is highly variable in accordance with factors such as the amount of alcohol consumed and the duration of exposure.

formal thought disorder: a core symptom of schizophrenia in which there is a disturbance in the logical connections between ideas. Features of formal thought disorder include poverty of (content of) speech, derailment and tangentiality.

fragile X syndrome: the most common inherited form of intellectual disability; caused by the fragile X mental retardation 1 (FMR1) gene on the X chromosome and more commonly seen in males.

frontotemporal dementia: a group of dementias which is associated with a range of neuropathologies including motor neurone disease, corticobasal degeneration, Pick's disease, progressive supranuclear palsy, Alzheimer's disease, Lewy body variant, prion disease and vascular dementia. Frontotemporal dementia includes a behavioural variant, semantic dementia and progressive non-fluent aphasia.

functional communication: verbal and nonverbal behaviours that express an individual's needs, wants, feelings and preferences with a view to being understood by others. For some clients with severe communication impairments, functional communication may be the goal of intervention.

functional voice disorder: *see* **dysphonia**

gastroesophageal reflux: *see* **laryngopharyngeal reflux**

gender dysphoria: also known as gender identity disorder, a condition in which a person experiences his or her phenotypic sex as incongruous with his or her sense of gender identity. Gender dysphoria can be treated through surgery (gender reassignment surgery), hormone treatment and voice therapy.

glomus jugulare tumour: a benign tumour which grows in the temporal bone of the skull in an area called the jugular foramen. The jugular vein and several important nerves exit the skull via the jugular foramen and these structures are at risk of damage from a tumour in this area. Symptoms include dysphagia, dizziness, hearing loss, pulsatile tinnitus, hoarseness, pain and facial nerve palsy.

glossectomy: surgical removal of the tongue, either in whole (total glossectomy) or in part (partial glossectomy), due to the presence of tongue cancer (primarily squamous cell carcinoma).

glossomania: a feature of schizophrenic language, also known as clanging, in which a speaker produces long sequences of utterances in which sound or meaning associations are developed.

Goldenhar's syndrome: also known as oculo-auriculo-vertebral dysplasia. A disorder of unknown aetiology, in which there is unilateral malformation of craniofacial structures, including eye, oral and musculoskeletal anomalies. Ear anomalies include auricular appendages, atresia of the external auditory canals (causing conductive hearing loss), unilateral microtia and unilateral posteriorly placed ear. Intellectual disability is not common in this syndrome.

granuloma: a benign, inflammatory lesion of the vocal folds which is most often located over the vocal process of the arytenoid cartilage. A corresponding ulcer is commonly found on the contralateral side. Granulomas tend to recur following surgical excision and have been linked to endotracheal intubation, gastroesophageal reflux, external laryngeal trauma and phonotrauma.

hemianopia: a visual field defect that is usually caused by strokes, head injuries and intracranial tumours. In homonymous hemianopia, there is loss of half of the visual field on one side in both eyes. This impairment can affect a variety of cognitive visual functions including reading, visual search and safe navigation through changing environments.

hemiplegia: a congenital or acquired condition in which there is paralysis of one side of the body. In a less serious condition known as hemiparesis, one side of the body is weak. Hemiplegia and hemiparesis are found in a number of the clinical groups managed by speech-language pathologists, including children with cerebral palsy and traumatic brain injury and adults with aphasia.

hyperadduction: a laryngeal finding in which there is increased closing force, or adduction time, in the glottal cycle. Hyperadduction can occur as a primary problem which may then give rise to secondary pathology. Alternatively, it may serve as a compensatory behaviour in response to the presence of laryngeal pathology. The speaker who engages in hyperadduction may have a vocal presentation which ranges from complete aphonia to a mildly hoarse voice.

hypernasality: excessive nasal resonance in speech which may be caused by velopharyngeal incompetence; a feature of cleft palate speech and dysarthric speech.

hypertonia: increased muscle tone. Hypertonia is a feature of some dysarthrias (e.g. spastic dysarthria) and neurodevelopmental disorders (e.g. cerebral palsy).

hyponasality: insufficient nasal resonance in speech which may be caused by enlarged adenoids and the presence of nasal polyps, amongst other things.

hypotonia: decreased muscle tone. Hypotonia is a feature of some dysarthrias (e.g. flaccid dysarthria) and certain syndromes (e.g. Prader-Willi syndrome).

intellectual disability: another term for mental retardation or learning disability; applies to children and adults with an intelligence quotient (IQ) below 70 such as occurs in a range of syndromes (e.g. Down's syndrome) and other clinical disorders (e.g. autism spectrum disorder).

intersex condition: a condition in which there is a discrepancy between the external genitalia and internal genitalia (testes and ovaries); includes Turner's syndrome, androgen insensitivity syndrome and congenital adrenal hyperplasia; an intersex condition must not be present for a diagnosis of gender identity disorder (gender dysphoria) to be made.

iteration: a speech feature of developmental stuttering in which a single speech sound or two speech sounds (the latter usually a schwa vowel) in syllable-initial or word-initial position is repeated, e.g. s-s-s-soap; sǝ-sǝ-sǝ-side.

jargon: a feature of fluent aphasia. Jargon can consist of English words linked together to produce meaningless utterances or the extensive use of neologisms in verbal output.

Kabuki make-up syndrome: a multiple congenital anomalies/mental retardation syndrome. The syndrome is characterized by a dysmorphic face, postnatal growth retardation, skeletal abnormalities, mild to moderate mental retardation and unusual dermatoglyphic patterns.

Landau-Kleffner syndrome: also known as acquired epileptic aphasia or aphasia with convulsive disorder; a rare disorder in which a child's language skills regress, either suddenly or gradually, in the presence of seizures.

laryngectomy: surgical removal of the larynx, either in whole (total laryngectomy) or in part (partial laryngectomy), due to the presence of laryngeal cancer; the person who undergoes this procedure is called a laryngectomee.

laryngitis: an acute or chronic inflammation of laryngeal tissues which results in vocal hoarseness. Laryngitis is most commonly caused by a viral infection. Less frequently, a bacterial infection may be the cause, necessitating antibiotic treatment. Vocal trauma and acid reflux are other possible causes of laryngitis.

laryngopharyngeal reflux: an extraoesophageal variant of gastroesophageal reflux disease that affects the larynx and pharynx. The acidic contents of the stomach make their way to the top of the oesophagus and spill over into the larynx. Laryngopharyngeal reflux has been linked to a number of vocal fold pathologies including laryngeal carcinoma.

laryngoscopy: a technique used to examine the larynx. In mirror laryngoscopy, the examining physician uses gauze to hold the end of the client's tongue while a laryngeal mirror is positioned just below the back of the soft palate as the patient says 'ee'. In patients where this procedure elicits a strong gag reflex, fibreoptic laryngoscopy may be a more appropriate technique. A flexible endoscope is passed transnasally into a position above the larynx. Insertion of the scope may be made more tolerable by the use of a local anaesthetic spray.

learning disability: the preferred term in the UK to refer to intellectual disability (q.v.); children and adults with learning disability have an intelligence quotient (IQ) of 70 or under; present in many syndromes (e.g. Down's syndrome) and other disorders (e.g. cerebral palsy).

Lewy body dementia: a form of dementia which shares clinical and pathological features with both Alzheimer's disease and Parkinson's disease. The condition is caused by the accumulation of Lewy bodies (aggregations of alpha-synuclein protein) inside the nuclei of neurones in certain regions of the brain. In dementia with Lewy bodies, deficits of attention, memory and executive function can be more severe than those found in Parkinson's disease dementia.

macroglossia: a condition in which the tongue is larger than normal; a feature of several syndromes including Down's syndrome and Beckwith-Wiedemann syndrome.

magnetic resonance imaging (MRI): a technique that employs a magnetic field and a radiofrequency pulse to create a magnetic resonance image. MRI has advantages over other imaging techniques. It is noninvasive, uses nonionizing radiation and produces high-quality images of soft tissue resolution in any imaging plane.

mandibulectomy: surgical removal of all or part of the mandible (lower jaw). This procedure may be performed during resection of primary tumours of the floor of the mouth when a tumour is either massive or directly invading the mandible.

mania: an abnormal and persistently elevated, expansive or irritable mood; this mood disturbance must be accompanied by other symptoms among which are included inflated self-esteem or grandiosity, psychomotor agitation, flight of ideas and pressure of speech.

maternal rubella: a viral infection which has severe consequences for a developing foetus. Although the rubella virus can affect the foetus at any stage of pregnancy, defects are rarely noted after the sixteenth week of gestation. The most common defects in the congenital rubella syndrome are hearing loss, intellectual disability, cardiac malformations and eye defects. The hearing loss is profound and sensorineural in nature.

Ménière's disease: an inner ear disorder in which the symptoms are tinnitus, vertigo and deafness; sensorineural hearing loss is low frequency and fluctuates.

meningitis: a bacterial or viral infection in which there is inflammation of the meninges, the membranes which envelope the brain and spinal cord; meningitis is a significant cause of developmental and acquired speech, language and hearing disorders.

mental retardation: *see* **intellectual disability**

microtia: a small, abnormally shaped or absent external ear or pinna that is present from birth. It is usually accompanied by a narrow, blocked or absent ear canal. Microtia can occur as an isolated clinical abnormality or as part of a syndrome (e.g. Goldenhar's syndrome).

Möbius syndrome: a rare neurological condition which affects the muscles that control facial expression and eye movement. Lesions of a number of the cranial nerves related to speech – trigeminal (V), facial (VII) and hypoglossal (XII) nerves – can produce a marked dysarthria.

motor neurone disease (MND): a progressive neurodegenerative disease in which there is a widespread and often rapid deterioration in upper and lower motor neurones. MND affects all aspects of speech production and eventually swallowing and feeding. There are three types of MND: amyotrophic lateral sclerosis, progressive bulbar palsy and progressive muscular atrophy.

multiple sclerosis: a neurodegenerative disease in which the myelin sheath which envelopes the axons of neurones is destroyed in a process known as demyelination. There are three types of multiple sclerosis: relapsing remitting, primary progressive and secondary progressive. Multiple sclerosis can cause dysarthria and swallowing problems. Increasingly, cognitive and language problems are being identified in this clinical population.

multiple subpial transection: a surgical procedure which is used in the treatment of Landau-Kleffner syndrome. Tangential, or horizontal, intracortical fibres are severed, while the vertical fibre connections of both incoming and outgoing nerve pathways are preserved. The selective disruption of neurones which have horizontal linkages eliminates the capacity of the treated cortex to produce epileptiform activity.

muscle tension dysphonia: also known as hyperfunctional voice disorder. A voice disorder in which there is a strained strangled voice quality which is similar to that of adductor spasmodic dysphonia. There is the appearance of excessive tension in the neck area and associated laryngeal hyperfunction. The patient frequently reports vocal fatigue.

muscular dystrophy: the most common neurological disorder after cerebral palsy to result in developmental dysarthria. All striated muscles, including those of the speech mechanism, atrophy and weaken in this disorder.

mutism: speechlessness, which can have a neurological or behavioural aetiology. Mutism is a feature of many clinical conditions including childhood posterior fossa tumour, traumatic brain injury, dementia and Landau-Kleffner syndrome.

myringotomy: a surgical procedure in which the otolaryngologist makes a small incision in the tympanic membrane, draws fluid out of the middle ear and inserts a ventilating or pressure equalizing tube; the procedure is used to treat recurrent episodes of otitis media.

nasal polyp: sac-like growths of inflamed tissue which line the nasal mucosa or sinuses. Polyps typically start near the ethmoid sinuses and grow into the open areas. Large polyps can block the nasal airway, resulting in hyponasal speech.

nasal regurgitation: the exiting of liquid and food from the nasal cavities during feeding. This condition is indicative of the presence of oronasal fistulae, velopharyngeal incompetence and/or clefts in the palate, all of which allow food and liquid to escape from the oral cavity into the nasal cavities. Nasal regurgitation can make feeding distressing and difficult for babies with cleft palate.

nasendoscopy: an investigative technique that involves passing a flexible tube (a scope) transnasally to a position above the velopharyngeal port. A local anaesthetic may be needed to make this invasive procedure tolerable for the client. Nasendoscopy allows clinicians to assess the function of the velopharyngeal mechanism.

nasometry: an objective technique which is used to measure the acoustic correlate of nasality. The nasometer produces a score which represents the ratio of energy in oral and nasal acoustic sound signals. Nasometry can be used to supplement the perception of hypernasal resonance in clients with velopharyngeal insufficiency.

neologism: means literally new ('neo') word ('logism'); neologisms are found in aphasia and schizophrenia (e.g. a schizophrenic speaker who utters 'geshinker').

noise-induced hearing loss: a reduction in hearing ability following exposure to loud sound may be temporary or permanent. With each episode of noise exposure, there is a noise-induced temporary threshold shift in hearing. Although there is recovery of hearing following these episodes, small amounts of permanent damage are also taking place. Permanent hearing loss arises when the swelling of the hair cells following noise exposure can lead to some cells rupturing. Hair cells may also become distorted, the stereocilia of these cells may fuse or may no longer transmit energy effectively to the hair cells.

oesophageal voice: a means of communication after laryngectomy in which the speaker swallows air into the oesophagus which is then vibrated in the oesophageal sphincter to produce voice.

oppositional defiant disorder (ODD): a childhood behavioural disorder; the fifth edition of the *Diagnostic and Statistical Manual of Mental Disorders* categorizes the symptoms of this disorder into three types: angry/irritable mood, argumentative/defiant behaviour, and vindictiveness. The frequency of these behaviours distinguishes the child or adolescent with ODD from normally developing children and adolescents, many of whom exhibit similar behaviours.

oral candidiasis: an opportunistic infection of the oral cavity which is caused by the yeast-like fungus candida (most often *Candida albicans*). Oral candidiasis is a common infection, particularly in certain groups (e.g. individuals with HIV infection).

organic voice disorder: *see* **dysphonia**

ossicular reconstruction: a surgical and prosthetic procedure used in the treatment of cholesteatoma which erodes the middle ear ossicles. When the cholesteatoma is removed, an ossicular reconstruction prosthesis, made of bone, teflon or stainless steel, is anchored between the eardrum and stapes footplate. Reconstruction may be partial or complete depending on how much of the original ossicular chain is replaced.

otitis media: an infection of the middle ear that is commonly known as 'glue ear'; otitis media can cause conductive hearing loss and repeated episodes can compromise speech development in children.

otoacoustic emissions testing: a technique which is used to test for the presence of sensorineural hearing loss in newborns. It is based on the observation that the cochlea can actually generate sounds (technically, emissions) either spontaneously (spontaneous otoacoustic emissions) or in response to acoustic stimulation (evoked otoacoustic emissions). These emissions are absent in mild inner ear deafness.

otolaryngologist: (also, otorhinolaryngologist) American term used to describe the medical specialist who assesses and treats ear, nose and throat disorders; known as an ENT specialist in the UK.

otosclerosis: a middle ear condition in which new bone growth on the anterior stapes footplate disrupts the functioning of the ossicular chain and causes conductive hearing loss; can be treated through a surgical procedure known as stapedectomy.

palilalia: a developmental or acquired disorder characterized by reiteration of utterances in the context of increasing rate (this feature is disputed by some) and decreasing loudness. The condition has been associated with bilateral subcortical neuropathology and developmental disorders such as autism.

papillomatosis: relatively rare, benign growths of the larynx that are caused by the human papilloma virus types 6 and 11. Papillomas grow quickly and can compromise the airway. They can also recur, necessitating repeated surgical interventions. Papillomas may cause inspiratory stridor, dyspnoea (laboured respiration) and hoarseness.

parkinsonian facies: a mask-like facial expression that is characteristic of patients with Parkinson's disease. The palpebral fissures (distance between upper and lower eyelids) are wider than normal and blinking is infrequent. Eyes have a staring appearance on account of these features, and because spontaneous ocular movements are lacking. The patient's facial muscles exhibit an unnatural immobility.

Parkinson's disease: a neurodegenerative disease which is caused by the loss of cells that produce dopamine (a neurotransmitter substance) in the substantia nigra of the brain. There are four forms of parkinsonism: idiopathic Parkinson's, multiple system atrophy, progressive supranuclear palsy and drug-induced parkinsonism. Dysarthria is commonly seen in Parkinson's disease with reduced vocal intensity a common and early feature of the disorder.

perseveration: the repetition of a linguistic form (word, phrase, etc.) beyond the point where it is appropriate; perseveration is a feature of the spoken output of several types of clients with communication disorders including adults with aphasia and patients with schizophrenia.

pervasive developmental disorder: *see* **autism spectrum disorder**

phenylketonuria: a rare, inherited condition in which an affected infant lacks an enzyme (phenylalanine hydroxylase) that is needed to break down the essential amino acid phenylalanine. The build-up of phenylalanine is harmful to the central nervous system and can cause brain damage.

phonemic paraphasia: a language error in which sounds are substituted, added or rearranged so that the uttered form has a sound resemblance to the target word (e.g. 'buckboard' for *cupboard*); a feature of aphasia in adults.

phonosurgery: a general term describing a range of surgical procedures that are intended to maintain or improve the quality of the voice by correcting defects in laryngeal sound production; includes laryngeal microsurgery (used to treat vocal nodules and polyps), medialization surgery (used to treat vocal fold paralysis), and cricothyroid approximation (used to achieve pitch elevation in male-to-female transsexuals).

Pierre Robin syndrome: this syndrome is characterized by micrognathia (severe underdevelopment of the mandible) and glossoptosis (falling back of the tongue) that causes airway obstruction and respiratory distress; approximately half of children with this syndrome can present with an incomplete cleft of the palate.

posterior fossa tumour: the posterior fossa is a small space in the skull which is found near the brainstem and cerebellum. The growth of a tumour in this area can block the flow of cerebrospinal fluid and increase pressure on the brain and spinal cord. Posterior fossa tumours account for half of all brain tumours in children. Mutism, dysarthria and dysphagia are associated with surgery for these tumours.

poverty of content of speech: spoken output which conveys little content or meaning despite being of an acceptable quantity or amount; a feature of schizophrenic language.

poverty of speech: also known as alogia; describes the substantially reduced verbal output that is a negative symptom of schizophrenia.

Prader-Willi syndrome: a deletion of the long arm of paternal chromosome 15 which is usually associated with mild intellectual disability. Individuals with this syndrome are distinguished by their voracious appetite (hyperphagia). Early, severe hypotonia can cause articulation problems, feeding difficulties and hypernasality due to velopharyngeal insufficiency. Language, particularly expressive language, is generally delayed.

pragmatic language impairment: a successor to the term 'semantic-pragmatic disorder'; describes a subgroup of children with SLI in which there are marked difficulties with the pragmatics of language.

preauricular pits and tags: tags are skin-coloured, fleshy appendages which appear as nodules or skin protrusions just in front of the tragus of the ear. Pits are depressions, dimples or fossae at the anterior margin of the ascending limb of the helix of the ear. Both pits and tags can be a feature of syndromes including oculo-auriculo-vertebral spectrum (both), oto-facio-cervical syndrome (pits) and Townes-Brocks syndrome (tags).

presbycusis: a condition in which there is deterioration of the cochlea and auditory nerve as a consequence of the natural aging process resulting in sensorineural hearing loss.

presbylarynx: literally 'old larynx', a voice disorder which is the result of degenerative, age-related changes in the larynx. In presbylarynx, the vocal folds close at the front and back but fail to adduct in the middle. This leads to a rapid loss of air through the glottis during phonation with consequent reduction of phonation time. Other glottic characteristics of presbylarynx include prominence of the vocal processes and a spindle-shaped glottic chink.

pressured speech: excessive speech which is produced at a rapid rate and is difficult to interrupt. It is one of the features of speech in hypomania and mania but rarely occurs in schizophrenia.

primary progressive aphasia (PPA): a slowly progressive aphasia which occurs initially in the absence of generalized dementia. As speech and language impairments in PPA worsen over time, patients begin to exhibit more of the classical symptoms of dementia. PPA is associated with a number of neuropathologies including Alzheimer's disease, frontotemporal dementia, Lewy body dementia and vascular dementia. Three subtypes of PPA are recognized: nonfluent/agrammatic, logopenic and semantic PPA.

prognosis: the probability or risk of an individual developing a particular state of health (an outcome) over a specific period of time given that individual's clinical and non-clinical profile. An outcome may include an event such as death or a quantity such as disease progression.

progressive non-fluent aphasia: a form of frontotemporal dementia in which a person's ability to produce fluent and grammatically well-formed speech is severely compromised. Agrammatism, effortful, slowed speech output, phonemic paraphasias and articulatory struggle are all present. Patients display difficulty comprehending syntactically complex sentences in the context of spared single-word comprehension and object knowledge. The condition evolves to complete mutism.

progressive supranuclear palsy: *see* **Parkinson's disease**

protraction: also known as perseveration; a speech feature of developmental stuttering in which a single speech sound is prolonged in syllable-initial or word-initial position, e.g. s::::soap.

psychosis: a condition in which there is a loss of contact with reality, delusions (the holding of false and bizarre beliefs) and hallucinations (the perception of things which do not exist). Psychosis is a feature of several mental illnesses including schizophrenia and bipolar disorder.

puberphonia: also known as mutational falsetto; typically seen in adolescent males who continue to speak with a pre-pubescent voice beyond the point at which voice mutation occurs.

pure tone audiometry: the most commonly performed hearing test, this pure tone air conduction procedure gives a record of hearing level by frequency (125 Hz–8 kHz). Sound is delivered to the ear canal via headphones or ear inserts and results are graphed on an audiogram.

recruitment: defined as the abnormally rapid growth of perceived loudness as intensity increases. Recruitment is thought to be a hallmark of cochlear dysfunction and is a feature of a number of disorders including presbycusis and Ménière's disease.

Reinke's oedema: also referred to as polypoid degeneration and polypoid corditis. This condition involves an expansion of Reinke's space by an inflammatory, gelatinous, amorphous material which extends from the anterior commissure to the vocal process. The swollen vocal folds prolapse inferiorly on inspiration, giving them a 'saddle bag' appearance.

right-hemisphere language disorder: stroke-induced and other lesions in the right hemisphere of the brain produce a different pattern of language impairment from that which occurs in left-hemisphere damage; while structural language is often intact, significant impairments in pragmatics and discourse can compromise many aspects of communication.

scanning speech: slow, deliberate, segmented, monotonous verbal output that is associated with cerebellar damage and is a feature of ataxic dysarthria. The prosodic features of rhythm and inflection are disrupted. Scanning speech may be found in advanced multiple sclerosis.

schizophrenia: a serious mental illness which is diagnosed on the basis of positive and negative symptoms; positive symptoms include thought disorder, delusions and hallucinations (mostly auditory); negative symptoms include affective flattening, poverty of speech, apathy, avolition and social withdrawal.

selective mutism: one of the emotional and behavioural disorders in which an affected child fails to communicate in a specific context (e.g. at school) despite doing so effectively in other contexts (e.g. at home); the failure to communicate is not on account of inadequate speech and language skills, although these may also be present.

semantic dementia: a form of frontotemporal dementia in which there is progressive bilateral degeneration of the temporal lobes. The most pronounced feature of this form of dementia is degradation of semantic knowledge which is evident across all modalities (e.g. written and spoken language) and modes of input and output (e.g. comprehension and expression).

semantic paraphasia: a language error in which a word that is semantically related to the target form is produced (e.g. 'ear' for *eye*); a feature of aphasia in adults.

sensorineural hearing loss: a hearing loss which is related to cochlear damage, impairment of the auditory pathway to the brain and damage of the auditory cortices in the brain; possible causes include infections such as meningitis, trauma and cerebrovascular accidents.

single-photon emission computed tomography (SPECT): a technique in which a radioactive drug is injected into a vein. A scanner makes detailed images of areas inside the body where the radioactive material is taken up by the cells. While SPECT has many applications in neurology and oncology, the majority of SPECT scans are performed in cardiology.

social communication: describes any form of communication the purpose of which is to establish, facilitate or maintain social relationships with others. Social communication depends on a range of linguistic and cognitive skills in the areas of pragmatics, social perception and social cognition.

spasmodic dysphonia: a neurogenic voice disorder consisting of adductor, abductor and mixed adductor-abductor types. In adductor spasmodic dysphonia, the most common type, the vocal folds spasm shut abruptly at irregular intervals during phonation. The symptoms of adductor spasmodic dysphonia are similar to those of muscle tension dysphonia, making a differential diagnosis difficult. The vocal folds fail to maintain normal contact during phonation in abductor spasmodic dysphonia.

specific language impairment (SLI): a severe developmental language disorder in children; SLI has been described as a diagnosis by exclusion as language impairment occurs in the absence of hearing loss, craniofacial anomaly, intellectual disability (i.e. a range of factors known to cause language disorder).

stapedectomy: surgical removal of the stapes, one of the middle ear ossicles. The stapes is replaced by a prosthesis. Stapedectomy is the treatment of choice for otosclerosis.

stenosis: a narrowing of a tubular structure or organ. Several types of stenosis are relevant to speech-language pathologists, including ear canal stenosis and subglottic stenosis (a narrowing of the airway below the vocal folds and above the trachea).

stridor: a harsh, vibratory sound of variable pitch which is caused by partial obstruction of the respiratory passages. Inspiratory stridor indicates obstruction of the airway above the glottis and is a symptom of many vocal fold pathologies. Expiratory stridor indicates obstruction in the lower trachea.

stroboscopy: a technique which is used to examine fine movement of the vocal folds and the mucosal wave. A microphone is placed on the neck of the patient. It allows the frequency of a strobe flashing light to be matched to the frequency of vocal fold vibration. The 'slow-motion' image is captured by a flexible endoscope or a 60° or 70° rigid telescope inserted into the mouth.

stroke: *see* **cerebrovascular accident**

stuttering: also known as stammering; a fluency disorder which is characterized by word- and syllable-initial iterations (repetitions) and perseverations (prolongations). Stuttering occurs in developmental, acquired (mostly neurogenic) and psychogenic forms.

sulcus vocalis: a linear depression or groove in the vocal fold mucosa which runs parallel to the free border and is usually bilateral and symmetrical. The glottic dysfunction in sulcus is complex, consisting of both glottal leakage (causing breathy voice) and stiffness of the free edge of the folds (causing rough voice).

surgical voice reconstruction: *see* **voice prosthesis**

theory of mind: the cognitive ability to attribute mental states (e.g. beliefs, knowledge) both to one's own mind and to the minds of others. Theory of mind deficits are a feature of many disorders in which there are significant communication problems including autism spectrum disorder and schizophrenia.

tinnitus: a roaring, buzzing or ringing sound in the ears which can impact on the mental health of affected individuals. Tinnitus is a symptom of many disorders including presbycusis, noise-induced hearing loss, ototoxicity related to the taking of aspirin and aminoglycoside antibiotics, Ménière's disease and acoustic neuroma.

Tourette's syndrome: a neurodevelopmental disorder in which an individual displays significant motor and phonic tics and coprophenomena (involuntary expression of socially unacceptable words or gestures). Researchers are beginning to identify speech, fluency and high-level language impairments in this clinical population.

tracheotomy: a surgical procedure in which a transverse or vertical incision is made into the trachea through the tissues of the neck in order to create a temporary or permanent opening for respiration. The procedure has a number of clinical applications including the long-term mechanical ventilation of patients.

traumatic brain injury: there are two forms of traumatic brain injury: in an open or penetrating head injury, the skull is fractured or otherwise breached by a missile; in a closed head injury, the brain is damaged while the skull remains intact.

Treacher Collins syndrome: a craniofacial syndrome in which there is hypoplasia of the zygomatic (cheek) bones and mandible (micrognathia), external ear abnormalities, notching of the lower eyelid and absence of lower eyelashes. Less commonly, cleft palate with or without cleft lip is present. Approximately half of individuals have a conductive hearing loss which is related to malformation of the ossicles and hypoplasia of the middle ear cavities.

Turner's syndrome: a syndrome which is caused by the absence of one of the X chromosomes (hence, the use of the terms XO syndrome, 45X syndrome and monosomy X for this disorder). The expression of the disorder is most severe in cases where there is a large percentage of body cells with a missing X chromosome. In such cases, there is an absence of secondary sexual characteristics, an absence of gonads and short stature. Individuals with this syndrome are also at risk for intellectual disability and communication disorders.

tympanometry: an objective technique for measuring the mobility or compliance of the tympanic membrane as a function of changing air pressures in the external auditory canal. This technique can be used to establish middle ear pressure through the measurement of the amount of air pressure in the external auditory canal that is needed to achieve maximum mobility of the eardrum.

varices or capillary ectasias: *see* **vocal fold haemorrhage**

velocardiofacial syndrome: a genetic disorder in which part of chromosome 22 is missing; features of this syndrome include cleft palate, heart defects, a characteristic facial appearance, minor learning problems, and speech and feeding problems.

velopharyngeal incompetence (VPI): the failure of the velopharyngeal port to close adequately during speech production; VPI can be caused by structural anomalies (e.g. a short velum or excessively capacious pharynx) or by neurological impairment (e.g. an immobile velum after a stroke).

videofluoroscopy: a radiological investigation in which fluoroscopic images appear on the monitor of an X-ray machine while a patient is swallowing a radio-opaque bolus. This procedure is used extensively in the assessment of swallowing and dysphagia, but may also be employed to understand aspects of articulation (e.g. velopharyngeal function).

vocal abuse and misuse: describes the many ways in which voice users can engage in phonatory behaviours (e.g. hyperadduction of vocal folds) and other practices (e.g. excessive occupational voice use) that put them at risk of developing a voice disorder.

vocal cyst: benign, vocal fold lesion which can be classified as an epidermic or mucous-retention cyst depending on its histological features. Epidermic cysts have a cavity with caseous content which is covered by stratified squamous epithelium which is often keratinized. Mucous cysts have mucous content and walls which are coated by a cylindrical ciliated epithelium.

vocal fold bowing: the failure of the vocal folds to approximate at the midline. Vocal fold bowing is a laryngeal finding in a number of voice disorders including presbylarynx, vocal fold paralysis and sulcus vocalis.

vocal fold haemorrhage: vocal folds may bleed or haemorrhage, causing tiny, visible capillaries (varices or capillary ectasias) or larger perfusions of blood into the tissue of the folds. Risk factors for vocal fold haemorrhage include phonotrauma, laryngeal trauma, aspirin, non-steroidal anti-inflammatories and hormonal imbalances.

vocal fold paralysis and paresis (VFPP): a significant cause of neurogenic voice disorder. In VFPP, the vocal folds do not adduct, abduct or elongate normally as a result of damage to one or more of the nerves that innervate them. Bilateral VFPP compromises the airway and necessitates a tracheotomy.

vocal nodule: small, benign growths that occur along the margins of the vocal folds mostly at the junction of the anterior and middle third of the fold. Nodules are the most common cause of voice disorders in school-age children and are often associated with professional voice users (e.g. singers). In both cases, these growths are the result of vocal abuse and misuse.

vocal polyp: a benign growth of the vocal fold which is larger than a vocal nodule. Polyps are fluid-filled and may have their own blood supply. Smoking, hypothyroidism, gastroesophageal reflux and vocal misuse are causes of polyps.

voice prosthesis: the use of a valve to produce voice in the client with a laryngectomy. The prosthesis is fitted, often at the time of laryngectomy, to permit the passage of the pulmonary airstream into the upper region of the oesophagus. When the client blocks the stoma, oesophageal voice is then achieved.

weak central coherence: a type of cognitive processing, typically seen in autism, in which there is a preference for parts over wholes. Applied to language, the child with autism may be unable to extract information from context and use it to make a global coherence inference about a character's action in a story.

Williams syndrome: a rare genetic disorder in which there is a deletion of 26 contiguous genes on chromosome 7q11.23; this genetic defect gives rise to intellectual disability and physical anomalies including dysmorphic facial features, elastin arteriopathy, short stature, connective tissue abnormalities and infantile hypercalcemia; the full-scale intelligence quotient is usually in the 50s to 60s with a range of 40–85.

Wilson's disease: also known as progressive lenticular degeneration and hepatolenticular degeneration. This is a rare, inherited, metabolic disorder in which the body is unable to process dietary copper. Copper is deposited most frequently in the brain, liver and cornea of the eye.

Typically, the disease has its onset between 6 and 40 years, but most often begins during the teenage years. Dysarthria and dysphagia are clinical features of Wilson's disease.

Wolf-Hirschhorn syndrome: a multiple malformation disorder caused by a deletion of a portion of the short arm of chromosome 4. The syndrome is characterized by abnormal craniofacial features, severe mental retardation, seizures, congenital heart malformations, microcephaly, failure to thrive and prenatal-onset growth retardation.

word-finding difficulty: an expressive language problem in which an individual cannot produce a target word and may substitute a vague term (e.g. thing, stuff) or engage in circumlocution (i.e. talk around the target word); a feature of many communication disorders including aphasia in adults.

Worster-Drought syndrome: also called congenital suprabulbar paresis, Worster-Drought syndrome is a type of cerebral palsy that results from lesion sites above the lower motor neurons in the brainstem. The syndrome affects the bulbar muscles (i.e. lips, tongue, soft palate, pharynx, larynx), which causes persistent difficulties with swallowing, feeding, speech, saliva control and airway protection.

References

Abusamra, V., Côté, H., Joanette, Y. and Ferreres, A. 2009. 'Communication impairments in patients with right hemisphere damage', *Life Span and Disability* **12**:1, 67–82.

Ackley, R. S. 2014. 'Hearing disorders', in L. Cummings (ed.), *Cambridge handbook of communication disorders*, Cambridge: Cambridge University Press, 359–80.

Alpern, C. S. 2010. 'Identification and treatment of Landau-Kleffner syndrome', *The ASHA Leader*, 21 September 2010.

Baker, J. 2003. 'Psychogenic voice disorders and traumatic stress experience: a discussion paper with two case reports', *Journal of Voice* **17**:3, 308–18.

Ball, M., Müller, N., Klopfenstein, M. and Rutter, B. 2009. 'The importance of narrow phonetic transcription for highly unintelligible speech: some examples', *Logopedics Phoniatrics Vocology* **34**:2, 84–90.

Barr, W. B., Bilder, R. M., Goldberg, E., Kaplan, E. and Mukherjee, S. 1989. 'The neuropsychology of schizophrenic speech', *Journal of Communication Disorders* **22**:5, 327–49.

Barry, W. J. and Timmermann, G. 1985. 'Mispronunciations and compensatory movements of tongue-operated patients', *British Journal of Disorders of Communication* **20**:1, 81–90.

Beeke, S., Wilkinson, R. and Maxim, J. 2007. 'Individual variation in agrammatism: a single case study of the influence of interaction', *International Journal of Language & Communication Disorders* **42**:6, 629–47.

Belenchia, P. and McCardle, P. 1985. 'Goldenhar's syndrome: a case study', *Journal of Communication Disorders* **18**:5, 383–92.

Biddle, K. R., McCabe, A. and Bliss, L. S. 1996. 'Narrative skills following traumatic brain injury in children and adults', *Journal of Communication Disorders* **29**:6, 447–69.

Bleile, K. 1982. 'Consonant ordering in Down's syndrome phonology', *Journal of Communication Disorders* **15**:4, 275–85.

Bliss, L. S., McCabe, A. and Miranda, A. E. 1998. 'Narrative assessment profile: discourse analysis for school-age children', *Journal of Communication Disorders* **31**:4, 347–63.

Bortolini, U. and Leonard, L. B. 2000. 'Phonology and children with specific language impairment: status of structural constraints in two languages', *Journal of Communication Disorders* **33**:2, 131–50.

Buckingham, H. W. and Rekart, D. M. 1979. 'Semantic paraphasia', *Journal of Communication Disorders* **12**:3, 197–209.

Chaika, E. 1982. 'A unified explanation for the diverse structural deviations reported for adult schizophrenics with disrupted speech', *Journal of Communication Disorders* **15**:3, 167–89.

Chaika, E. and Alexander, P. 1986. 'The ice cream stories: a study of normal and psychotic narrations', *Discourse Processes* **9**:3, 305–28.

Chaika, E. and Lambe, R. A. 1989. 'Cohesion in schizophrenic narratives, revisited', *Journal of Communication Disorders* **22**:6, 407–21.

Chapman, S. B., Highley, A. P., and Thompson, J. L. 1998. 'Discourse in fluent aphasia and Alzheimer's disease: linguistic and pragmatic considerations', *Journal of Neurolinguistics* **11**:1–2, 55–78.

Chin, S. B., Finnegan, K. R. and Chung, B. A. 2001. 'Relationships among types of speech intelligibility in pediatric users of cochlear implants', *Journal of Communication Disorders* **34**:3, 187–205.

Clegg, J., Brumfitt, S., Parks, R. W. and Woodruff, P. W. R. 2007. 'Speech and language therapy intervention in schizophrenia: a case study', *International Journal of Language & Communication Disorders* **42**:S1, 81–101.

Conroy, P., Sage, K. and Ralph, M. L. 2009. 'Improved vocabulary production after naming therapy in aphasia: can gains in picture naming generalise to connected speech?', *International Journal of Language & Communication Disorders* **44**:6, 1036–62.

Cummings, L. 2008. *Clinical linguistics*, Edinburgh: Edinburgh University Press.

2009. *Clinical pragmatics*, Cambridge: Cambridge University Press.

2011. 'Pragmatic disorders and their social impact', *Pragmatics and Society* **2**:1, 17–36.

2012. 'Pragmatic disorders', in H.-J. Schmid (ed.), *Cognitive pragmatics* [Handbook of Pragmatics, Vol. 4], Berlin and Boston: Walter de Gruyter, 291–315.

2013a. 'Clinical linguistics: a primer', *International Journal of Language Studies* **7**:2, 1–30.

2013b. 'Clinical pragmatics and theory of mind', in A. Capone, F. Lo Piparo and M. Carapezza (eds.), *Perspectives on linguistic pragmatics*, Perspectives in Pragmatics, Philosophy and Psychology, Vol. 2, Dordrecht: Springer, 23–56.

2014a. *Communication disorders*, Houndmills: Palgrave Macmillan.

2014b. 'Clinical pragmatics', in Y. Huang (ed.), *Oxford handbook of pragmatics*, Oxford: Oxford University Press, to appear.

2014c. 'Pragmatic disorders and theory of mind', in L. Cummings (ed.), *Cambridge handbook of communication disorders*, Cambridge: Cambridge University Press, 559–77.

2014d. *Pragmatic disorders*, Dordrecht: Springer.

Dabul, B. 2000. *Apraxia battery for adults*, second edition, Austin, TX: Pro-Ed.

Dalemans, R. J. P., de Witte, L., Wade, D. and van den Heuvel, W. 2010. 'Social participation through the eyes of people with aphasia', *International Journal of Language & Communication Disorders* **45**:5, 537–50.

Day, L. S. and Parnell, M. M. 1987. 'Ten-year study of a Wilson's disease dysarthric', *Journal of Communication Disorders* **20**:3, 207–18.

Dorman, M. F., Sharma, A., Gilley, P., Martin, K. and Roland, P. 2007. 'Central auditory development: evidence from CAEP measurements in children fitted with cochlear implants', *Journal of Communication Disorders* **40**:4, 284–94.

Dronkers, N. F. 1996. 'A new brain region for coordinating speech articulation', *Nature* **384**: 159–61.

Fine, J. 2006. *Language in psychiatry: a handbook of clinical practice*, London: Equinox Publishing.

Gallena, S. K. 2007. *Voice and laryngeal disorders: a problem-based clinical guide with voice samples*, St Louis, MO: Mosby Elsevier.

Goldstein, B. A. and Iglesias, A. 1996. 'Phonological patterns in Puerto Rican Spanish-speaking children with phonological disorders', *Journal of Communication Disorders* **29**:5, 367–87.

Goodglass, H., Kaplan, E. and Barresi, B. 2001. *Boston diagnostic aphasia examination*, third edition, Baltimore, MD: Lippincott Williams & Wilkins.

Goss, J. 2006. 'The poetics of bipolar disorder', *Pragmatics & Cognition* **14**:1, 83–110.

Grunwell, P. and Huskins, S. 1979. 'Intelligibility in acquired dysarthria – a neuro-phonetic approach: three case studies', *Journal of Communication Disorders* **12**:1, 9–22.

Harris, J. and Cottam, P. 1985. 'Phonetic features and phonological features in speech assessment', *British Journal of Disorders of Communication* **20**:1, 61–74.

Horton, S., Byng, S., Bunning, K. and Pring, T. 2004. 'Teaching and learning speech and language therapy skills: The effectiveness of classroom as clinic in speech and language therapy student education', *International Journal of Language & Communication Disorders* **39**:3, 365–90.

Hough, M. S. 1993. 'Treatment of Wernicke's aphasia with jargon: a case study', *Journal of Communication Disorders* **26**:2, 101–11.

Howard, S. J. 1993. 'Articulatory constraints on a phonological system: a case study of cleft palate speech', *Clinical Linguistics & Phonetics* **7**:4, 299–317.

Joanette, Y., Ska, B. and Côté, H. 2004. *Protocole Montréal d'evaluation de la communication (MEC)*, Isbergues, France: Ortho-Édition.

Kent, R. D., Weismer, G., Kent, J. F. and Rosenbek, J. C. 1989. 'Toward phonetic intelligibility testing in dysarthria', *Journal of Speech and Hearing Disorders* **54**:4, 482–99.

Kristoffersen, K. E. 2008. 'Consonants in cri du chat syndrome: a case study', *Journal of Communication Disorders* **41**:3, 179–202.

La Pointe, L. L. and Johns, D. F. 1975. 'Some phonemic characteristics in apraxia of speech', *Journal of Communication Disorders* **8**:3, 259–69.

Leder, S. B. 1996. 'Adult onset of stuttering as a presenting sign in a Parkinsonian-like syndrome: a case report', *Journal of Communication Disorders* **29**:6, 471–8.

Lenden, J. M. and Flipsen Jr, P. 2007. 'Prosody and voice characteristics of children with cochlear implants', *Journal of Communication Disorders* **40**:1, 66–81.

Loukusa, S., Leinonen, E., Jussila, K., Mattila, M.-L., Ryder, N., Ebeling, H. and Moilanen, I. 2007. 'Answering contextually demanding questions: pragmatic errors produced by children with Asperger syndrome or high-functioning autism', *Journal of Communication Disorders* **40**:5, 357–81.

Mackay, L. and Hodson, B. 1982. 'Phonological process identification of misarticulations of mentally retarded children', *Journal of Communication Disorders* **15**:3, 243–50.

Marquardt, T. P., Jacks, A. and Davis, B. L. 2004. 'Token-to-token variability in developmental apraxia of speech: three longitudinal case studies', *Clinical Linguistics & Phonetics* **18**:2, 127–44.

Marshall, J. 2009. 'Framing ideas in aphasia: the need for thinking therapy', *International Journal of Language & Communication Disorders* **44**:1, 1–14.

Martins, R. H. G., Silva, R., Ferreira, D. M. and Dias, N. H. 2007. 'Sulcus vocalis: probable genetic etiology. Report of four cases in close relatives', *Brazilian Journal of Otorhinolaryngology* **73**:4, 573.

McCabe, P. J., Sheard, C. and Code, C. 2008. 'Communication impairment in the AIDS dementia complex (ADC): a case report', *Journal of Communication Disorders* **41**:3, 203–22.

McCardle, P. and Wilson, B. 1993. 'Language and development in FG syndrome with callosal agenesis', *Journal of Communication Disorders* **26**:2, 83–100.

McNeill, B. C. and Gillon, G. T. 2011. 'Prospective evaluation of features of childhood apraxia of speech', American Speech-Language-Hearing Association (ASHA) Convention: San Diego, CA, 17–19 November 2011.

Moore, M. E. 2001. 'Third person pronoun errors by children with and without language impairment', *Journal of Communication Disorders* **34**:3, 207–28.

Mount, K. H. and Salmon, S. J. 1988. 'Changing the vocal characteristics of a postoperative transsexual patient: a longitudinal study', *Journal of Communication Disorders* **21**:3, 229–38.

Mower, D. E. and Younts, J. 2001. 'Sudden onset of excessive repetitions in the speech of a patient with multiple sclerosis: a case report', *Journal of Fluency Disorders* **26**:4, 269–309.

Myers, P. S. 1979. 'Profiles of communication deficits in patients with right cerebral hemisphere damage: implications for diagnosis and treatment', *Clinical Aphasiology Conference*, Phoenix: BRK Publishers, 38–46.

Neuman, A., Molinelli, P. and Hochberg, I. 1981. 'Post-meningitic hearing loss: report on three cases', *Journal of Communication Disorders* **14**:2, 105–11.

Nowak, C. B. 1998. 'Genetics and hearing loss: a review of Stickler syndrome', *Journal of Communication Disorders* **31**:5, 437–54.

Oller, D. K., Jensen, H. T. and Lafayette, R. H. 1978. 'The relatedness of phonological processes of a hearing-impaired child', *Journal of Communication Disorders* **11**:2–3, 97–105.

Orange, J. B., Kertesz, A. and Peacock, J. 1998. 'Pragmatics in frontal lobe dementia and primary progressive aphasia', *Journal of Neurolinguistics* **11**:1–2, 153–77.

Pascoe, M., Stackhouse, J. and Wells, B. 2005. 'Phonological therapy within a psycholinguistic framework: promoting change in a child with persisting speech difficulties', *International Journal of Language & Communication Disorders* **40**:2, 189–220.

Peets, K. F. 2009. 'Profiles of dysfluency and errors in classroom discourse among children with language impairment', *Journal of Communication Disorders* **42**:2, 136–54.

Prinz, P. M. 1980. 'A note on requesting strategies in adult aphasics', *Journal of Communication Disorders* **13**:1, 65–73.

Santos, V. J. B., Mattioli, F. M., Mattioli, W. M., Daniel, R. J. and Cruz, V. P. M. 2006. 'Laryngeal dystonia: case report and treatment with botulinum toxin', *Brazilian Journal of Otorhinolaryngology* **72**:3, 425–7.

Scaler Scott, K. 2014. 'Stuttering and cluttering', in L. Cummings (ed.), *Cambridge handbook of communication disorders*, Cambridge: Cambridge University Press, 341–58.

Schuele, C. M. and Dykes, J. C. 2005. 'Complex syntax acquisition: a longitudinal case study of a child with specific language impairment', *Clinical Linguistics & Phonetics* **19**:4, 295–318.

Sebastian, C. L., Fontaine, N. M. G., Bird, G., Blakemore, S.-J., De Brito, S. A., McCrory, E. J. P. and Viding, E. 2012. 'Neural processing associated with cognitive and affective theory of mind in adolescents and adults', *Social Cognitive and Affective Neuroscience* **7**:1, 53–63.

Semel, E., Wiig, E. H. and Secord, W. A. 2003. *Clinical evaluation of language fundamentals*, fourth edition, Australia: Psychological Corporation.

Shanmugiah, A., Sinha, S., Taly, A. B., Prashanth, L. K., Tomar, M., Arunodaya, G. R., Reddy, J. Y. C. and Khanna, S. 2008. 'Psychiatric manifestations in Wilson's disease: a cross-sectional analysis', *The Journal of Neuropsychiatry and Clinical Neurosciences* **20**:1, 81–5.

Smith, C. R. 1975. 'Interjected sounds in deaf children's speech', *Journal of Communication Disorders* **8**:2, 123–8.

Smith, R. J. H. and Schwartz, C. 1998. 'Branchio-oto-renal syndrome', *Journal of Communication Disorders* **31**:5, 411–21.

Stribling, P., Rae, J. and Dickerson, P. 2007. 'Two forms of spoken repetition in a girl with autism', *International Journal of Language & Communication Disorders* **42**:4, 427–44.

Temple, C. 1997. *Developmental cognitive neuropsychology*, Hove: Psychology Press.

Temple, C. M. 1988. 'Developmental dyslexia and dysgraphia persistence in middle age', *Journal of Communication Disorders* **21**:3, 189–207.

Van Borsel, J. 1988. 'An analysis of the speech of five Down's syndrome adolescents', *Journal of Communication Disorders* **21**:5, 409–21.

Van Borsel, J., De Cuypere, G., Rubens, R. and Destaerke, B. 2000. 'Voice problems in female-to-male transsexuals', *International Journal of Language & Communication Disorders* **35**:3, 427–42.

Van Borsel, J., De Grande, S., Van Buggenhout, G. and Fryns, J.-P. 2004. 'Speech and language in Wolf-Hirschhorn syndrome: a case-study', *Journal of Communication Disorders* **37**:1, 21–33.

Van Lancker Sidtis, D. 2004. 'When novel sentences spoken or heard for the first time in the history of the universe are not enough: toward a dual-process model of language', *International Journal of Language & Communication Disorders* **39**:1, 1–44.

Van Lierde, K. M., Van Borsel, J. and Van Cauwenberge, P. 2000. 'Speech patterns in Kabuki make-up syndrome: a case report', *Journal of Communication Disorders* **33**:6, 447–62.

Ward, D. 2006. *Stuttering and cluttering: frameworks for understanding and treatment*, Hove: Psychology Press.

Wolk, L. and Edwards, M. L. 1993. 'The emerging phonological system of an autistic child', *Journal of Communication Disorders* **26**:3, 161–77.

Yaruss, J. S. 2014. 'Disorders of fluency', in L. Cummings (ed.), *Cambridge handbook of communication disorders*, Cambridge: Cambridge University Press, 484–97.

Yavas, M. and Hernandorena, C. M. 1991. 'Systematic sound preference in phonological disorders: a case study', *Journal of Communication Disorders* **24**:2, 79–87.

Index